A Beautiful Life: Forgotten Phyllis

Our Family's Battle with the Scourge of Alzheimer's

Raleigh Coffin

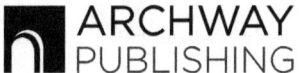

Copyright © 2018 Raleigh Coffin.

All rights reserved. No part of this book may be used or reproduced by any means, graphic, electronic, or mechanical, including photocopying, recording, taping or by any information storage retrieval system without the written permission of the author except in the case of brief quotations embodied in critical articles and reviews.

Archway Publishing books may be ordered through booksellers or by contacting:

Archway Publishing
1663 Liberty Drive
Bloomington, IN 47403
www.archwaypublishing.com
1 (888) 242-5904

Because of the dynamic nature of the Internet, any web addresses or links contained in this book may have changed since publication and may no longer be valid. The views expressed in this work are solely those of the author and do not necessarily reflect the views of the publisher, and the publisher hereby disclaims any responsibility for them.

Any people depicted in stock imagery provided by Getty Images are models, and such images are being used for illustrative purposes only. Certain stock imagery © Getty Images.

ISBN: 978-1-4808-6124-4 (sc)
ISBN: 978-1-4808-6123-7 (hc)
ISBN: 978-1-4808-6125-1 (e)

Library of Congress Control Number: 2018905606

Print information available on the last page.

Archway Publishing rev. date: 06/13/2018

I have recently been told that I am one of the millions of Americans who will be afflicted with Alzheimer's disease. I now begin the journey that will lead me into the sunset of my life. I know that for America there will always be a bright dawn ahead.

—President Ronald W. Reagan
November 5, 1994

It really is the long, long goodbye.

—Nancy Reagan
2002

Contents

Preface ix

The Seven Stages of Alzheimer's Disease 1
What Is Alzheimer's Disease? 6
Us 12
Mild-Early Stage 1 19
Respite 21
The Ten Nevers 25
Driving 28
Caregivers 33
Full-Time Home Care 39
Nursing Home Types 42
Long-Term Care 53
Moderate Stage 2 58
Remote Family and Friends 62
Advanced Stage 3 67
Finances 72
Financial Alternatives 80
Nursing Home I 87
Nursing Home II (Memory Care) 92
Nursing Home III (Memory Care) 96

Nursing Home IV (Rehab) 100
Nursing Home V (Private Home Care) 109
Death—Hospice 112
Loss 119
My Funeral Comments 126

Appendix A: Medical Advances 131
Appendix B: Diet 141
Appendix C: Medical Directives 151
References 159
Afterword 163
In Appreciation 167

Preface

Although this is a personal story, the experiences described within are not unique to me, Phyllis, or our family. At this point in time, the exact cause of the disease is not known. It is believed that the disease is caused by one or both distinctive proteins present in the brains of Alzheimer's patients.

This is not a story with a happy ending; its purpose is, through my own experience, to familiarize others with the disease and its personal impact on patient, caregiver, and family. I also describe various forms Alzheimer's disease can take and provide a few suggestions for coping with the "long goodbye."

This book is also not an ultimate resource book or a problem-solving guide, but it might help the afflicted and families anticipate some of the manifestations and symptoms of the disease.

There are many forms of dementia, and Alzheimer's constitutes about 80 percent of these cases. Although much of dementia carries the Alzheimer's label, the symptoms, duration, behaviors, and rates of the decline can vary greatly as can the types of diagnosis, medication, and caregiving.

This is also not a how-to book, although I will pass on some of the advice and knowledge that was provided to me by doctors, nurses, other victims, other caregivers, assisted living facilities, and memory care units. In this book, I will be talking primarily to the caregiver/family members and dwell to some extent on the role and challenges of the caregivers—professional, family, or institution. Since caregiving is perhaps one of the most devastating, demanding, and time-consuming aspects of the disease, it bears attention and discussion.

I will also provide some comments on dealing with finances, costs, insurance, health directives, and grimly, but importantly, "end-of-life" decisions associated with the disease. For me, they provided another impact or layer of worry; I never expected the amounts of administration and paperwork that were generated in part by the tasks above. They are ongoing and bleed into the grieving process.

There are three recognized stages of Alzheimer's, according to the medical profession, plus end of life:

- mild-early stage
- moderate stage

- severe-late stage
- death

The lines between these arbitrary stages are somewhat blurred, and an Alzheimer's disease patient may have some stage 2 symptoms while being basically still in stage 1. Also, there are no hard and set rules for the amount of time individuals pass through the stages. In fact, the list below expands the stages and shows seven distinct phases as provided by Massachusetts General Hospital.

The Seven Stages of Alzheimer's Disease

Stage 1: No Impairment

During this stage, Alzheimer's disease is not detectable, and no memory problems or other symptoms of dementia are evident.

Stage 2: Very Mild Decline

The senior may notice minor memory problems or lose things around the house—although not to the point where the memory loss can easily be distinguished from normal age-related memory loss. The person will still do well on memory tests, and the disease is unlikely to be detected by physicians or loved ones.

Stage 3: Mild Decline

At this stage, the friends and family members of the care receiver may begin to notice memory and cognitive problems. Performance on memory and cognitive tests will decline, and physicians will be able to detect impaired cognitive function. Patients in stage 3 will have difficulty in many areas, including:

- finding the right word during conversations
- remembering names of new acquaintances
- planning and organizing

People with stage 3 Alzheimer's may also frequently lose personal possessions, including valuables.

Stage 4: Moderate Decline

In this stage of Alzheimer's disease, clear-cut symptoms of Alzheimer's disease are apparent. Patients with stage 4 Alzheimer's disease:

- have difficulty with simple arithmetic
- may forget details about their life histories
- have poor short-term memory (may not recall what they ate for breakfast, for example)
- are not able to manage finances and pay bills

Stage 5: Moderately Severe Decline

During the fifth stage of Alzheimer's, patients begin to need help with many day-to-day activities. People in this stage of the disease may experience:

- significant confusion
- inability to recall simple details about themselves, such as their own phone number
- difficulty dressing appropriately

On the other hand, patients in this stage still maintain a modicum of functionality. They typically can still bathe and toilet independently. They also usually still know their family members and some details about their personal histories, especially their childhood and youth.

Stage 6: Severe Decline

Patients at this stage of Alzheimer's disease need constant supervision and frequently require professional care. Symptoms include:

- confusion or unawareness of environment and surroundings
- major personality changes and potential behavior problems
- the need for assistance with activities of daily living such as toileting, eating, and bathing
- inability to recognize faces except closest friends and relatives
- inability to remember most details of personal history
- loss of bowel and bladder control

- wandering

Stages 7: Very Severe Decline

This is the final stage of Alzheimer's disease. Because Alzheimer's disease is a terminal illness, patients in stage 7 are nearing death. In stage 7 of the disease, patients lose the ability to respond to their environment or communicate. While they may still be able to utter words and phrases, they have no insight into their condition and need assistance with all activities of daily living. In the final stages of the illness, patients may lose the ability to swallow, and their muscles will not function properly. Fortunately, as in the case of my wife, Phyllis, many patients succumb to less torturous endings, such as pneumonia, malnutrition, or stroke.

Notes

What Is Alzheimer's Disease?

Alzheimer's is a progressive and eventually fatal disease that was identified as early as 1906 by Dr. Alois Alzheimer, a Bavarian neuropathologist and psychiatrist. At this point in time, we believe that the disease is due to clusters in the brain consisting of protein fragments, called amyloid plaques that build up between nerve cells, eventually destroying all cognitive activity. The exact cause of the disease is not known. Besides amyloid proteins, neurofibrillary tangles (tau) are also present. Science has yet to determine the interrelationship or measure the impact of these two damaging proteins and how to prevent their formation.

Alzheimer's disease predominately appears in individuals over sixty years of age, and up until very recently, it was only truly distinguished from dementia by a postmortem autopsy. Alzheimer's disease results in gradual memory loss and other cognitive abnormalities over time that seriously interfere with daily life and day-to-day functioning. In addition to loss of memory, Alzheimer's disease can also be manifested by disorientation, language problems, judgment, and behavior changes such as anger, mood, perspective, and activity level. Things we take for granted today, such as preparing meals, driving, household chores, paying bills, and eventually conversation, recognition, and orientation disappear over time until the victim of the disease needs 24/7 care. Alzheimer's disease affects about 5.4 million Americans, which means that twenty to twenty-five million family members and friends are involved to some degree with the victims.

Grim as this picture is, there is some good news in that earlier detection is now possible. There are hundreds of human tests underway (see "Medical Advances"), and some of them look quite promising. Meanwhile, medical breakthroughs have not been a success with a 99 percent failure rate, meaning the availability of a "cure" could be quite a ways off, which brings us to dealing with the disease itself.

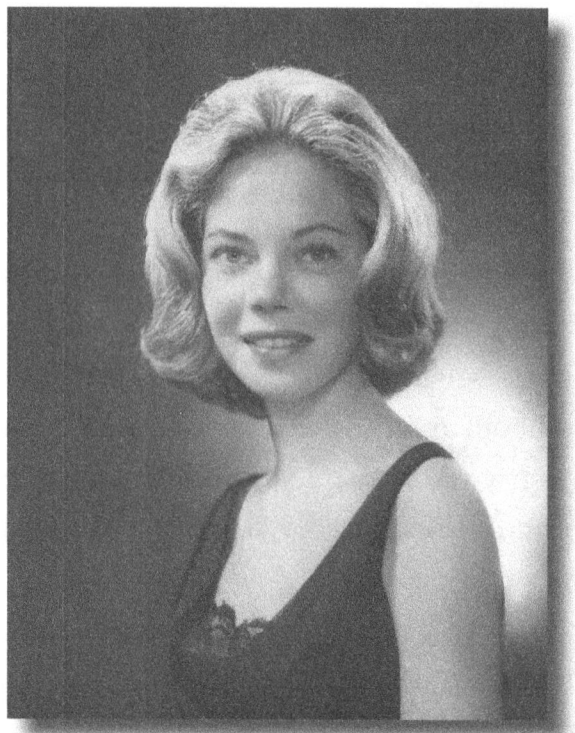

Phyllis Claire Verkamp (Engagement Picture)

After graduating from Yale in the late 1950s, I went to work in Procter & Gamble's marketing department in Cincinnati, Ohio. At one of the first parties I went to, I danced briefly with a beautiful girl named Phyllis Verkamp. At that juncture, we did little more than exchange names. I ran into her a few times over the next year, but we just talked briefly.

In 1959, my third year with P&G, I saw her picture in the local paper under the heading "Beautiful Faces in Beautiful Places," which informed me that she was spending her junior year at the University of London. The following year, after her graduation from Marymount College, I ran into her at a political rally at the Cincinnati airport where she and other local girls were acting as cheerleaders. After the rally, I offered her a ride home, which she accepted principally because I had a convertible with the top down, and she could wave her pom-poms. I offered her a cocktail at a local bar when we got to town, which she accepted, and we chatted for quite a while.

Toward the end, I asked her out on a date to which she agreed, but she warned me that she was returning to San Francisco to live after spending the holidays with her family in Cincinnati.

We dated several times, and just after Christmas, we had our "last date ever" since she was returning to San Francisco for New Year's Day. It really wasn't until she left that I realized I was in love with this beautiful girl who combined a sense of humor, kindness, and amazingly strong spirituality. She was a devoted Catholic and attended Mass regularly. I was even impressed by her family; they seemed to be very cohesive and loving and jokingly referred to me as a "non-Catholic." My last words to her (I thought) were: "Phyllis, have a good life!"

At our fiftieth wedding anniversary in 2013, I told this story to my assembled family and friends and thanked God that she had returned from San Francisco the following summer.

Notes

Us

Looking back over the years of marriage, the Coffin family had indeed been a very lucky one. We had lived in nice houses, generally on the water, and our kids were not too troublesome. They attended private schools, completed college, and found work. Without their mother as a mainstay and a moral compass, things might've been different.

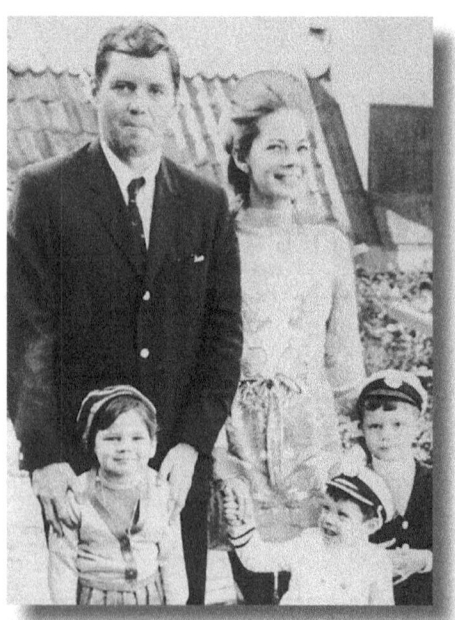

The Coffin Family in Sweden

Phyllis

During my career, we lived in several countries (Sweden, Spain, Italy, and Brazil). In each case, Phyllis had to move homes, find schools for the children, adapt to the language, and keep the kids motivated and centered. All this she did in style and cheerfully.

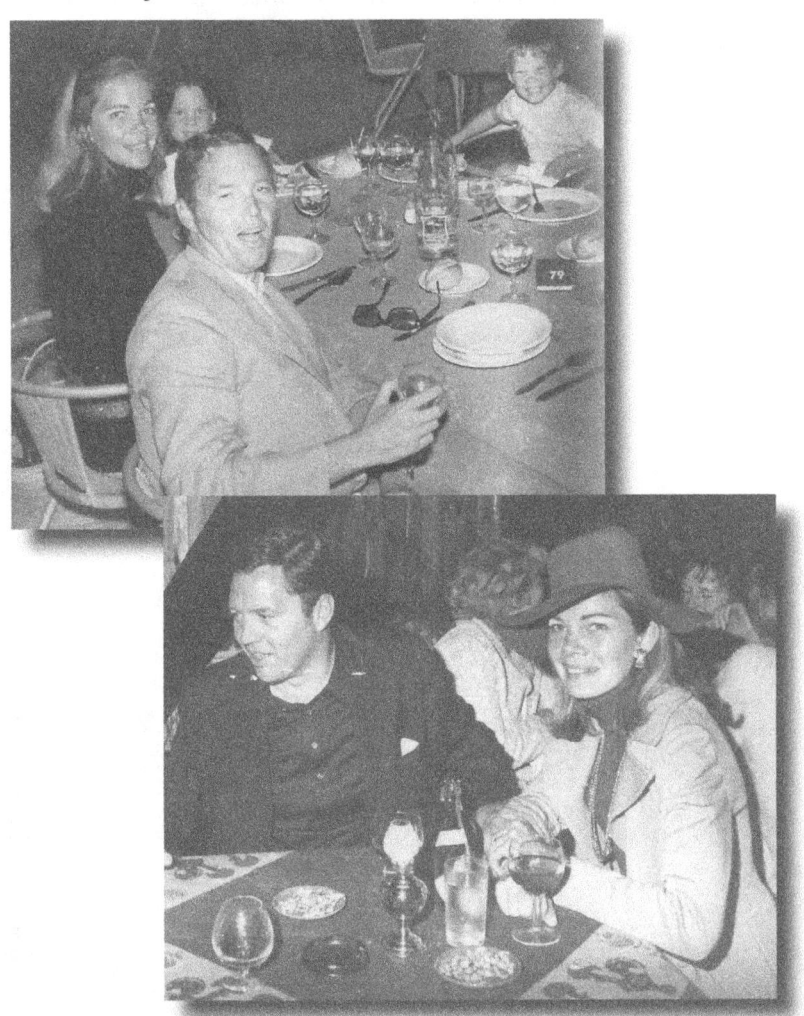

The Coffins in Spain

Phyllis had made it clear before we were married that her children would be raised Catholic, which I applauded since I thought it was much more likely that she would be going to church on Sunday mornings than I would. And she did. She took the children with her and brought them up with strong Christian values and love.

In 2002, after forty years of marriage, my sixty-four-year-old wife and I decided to pull up stakes from our house on Long Island Sound in Old Greenwich, Connecticut, and rent a condo on the ocean in Vero Beach, Florida, for the winter months.

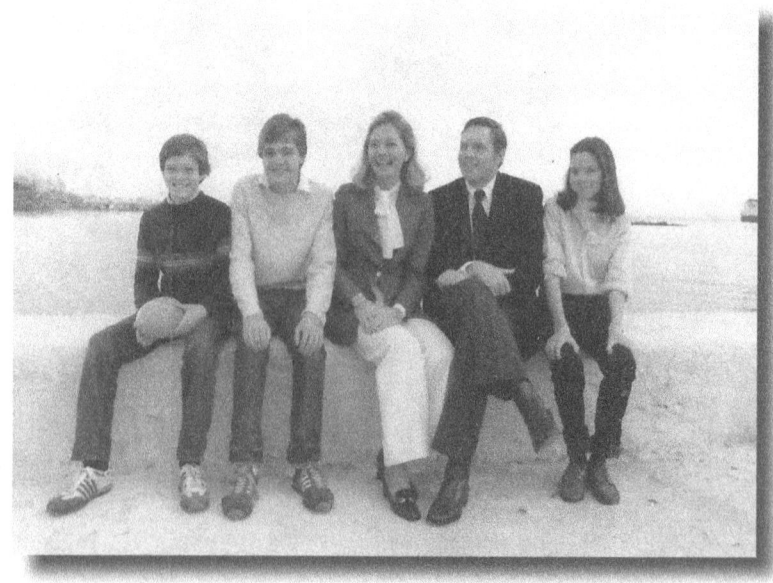

On Our Sea Wall in Old Greenwich

We eventually sold our Connecticut home and bought a house in Vero Beach. We planned to return to Connecticut each summer and rent near our three grown children, who were all in the tristate area.

Since we retained our Connecticut affiliations, golf, swimming, and boating were available to us, and we were also near the kids. I had fully retired from a career with major consumer products and entertainment corporations (P&G, Nabisco brands, Kraft/General Foods, and CBS/Fox).

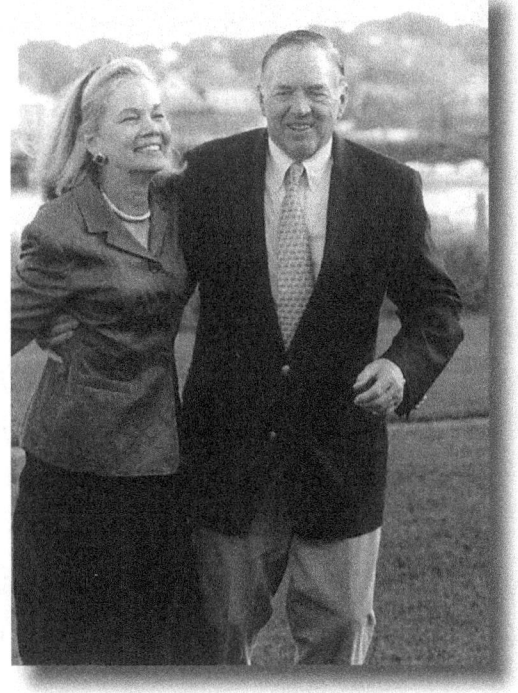

Phyllis and Raleigh

Phyllis was an extremely healthy person (no smoking or drinking), and she read just about every book on health—both allopathic and alternative. She collected extensive articles and newsletters on health. In the fifty years I'd known her, her weight had been constant, and she had kept her youthful good looks.

At a recent college reunion, a classmate asked me if she were a trophy wife—assuming she was at least twenty years younger than me (actually she was five).

I had always assumed that I would predecease Phyllis by ten or twenty years, and it was only to support her in my dotage that I bought a long-term-care policy for us both. Phyllis's continuing exploration of alternative medicine helped me over a few bumps. I loved ocean swimming at our small beach house in the Hamptons. One day, I had terrific pain in my foot and toes after a swim. I assumed I had been bitten by something in the ocean. Before the doctor even examined me the next day, his nurse handed me a brochure on gout. This was kind of annoying and presumptuous of the nurse until the doctor confirmed the gout and said I would be on medication for the rest of my life in order to control my uric acid levels.

Phyllis

Phyllis, who was not a big fan of prescription medicines, said, "Taking this lifetime medication is ridiculous." She put me on a diet of concentrated black cherry juice that "conquered" my gout in a day or two. She also once "cured" me from a bout of hepatitis by giving me voluminous amounts of vitamin C. The doctor was so amazed at my recovery that he preferred to say he provided the wrong diagnoses rather than admit that the vitamin medication had actually worked.

She was so healthy that I was somewhat perplexed when, in 2004 and 2005, she started misplacing things, forgetting names, and had trouble articulating a complete sentence. Just before our fiftieth anniversary celebration in Vero Beach in 2006, the doctors confirmed that she had "dementia of the Alzheimer's type." This began my exploration of the disease and the dramatic changes in my life as I transitioned from husband to caregiver.

Consequently, it was with an almost unfathomable sense of loss to see her slipping away each day over the estimated ten years of affliction as her body and mind were eroded by the onslaught of Alzheimer's disease.

Notes

Mild-Early Stage 1

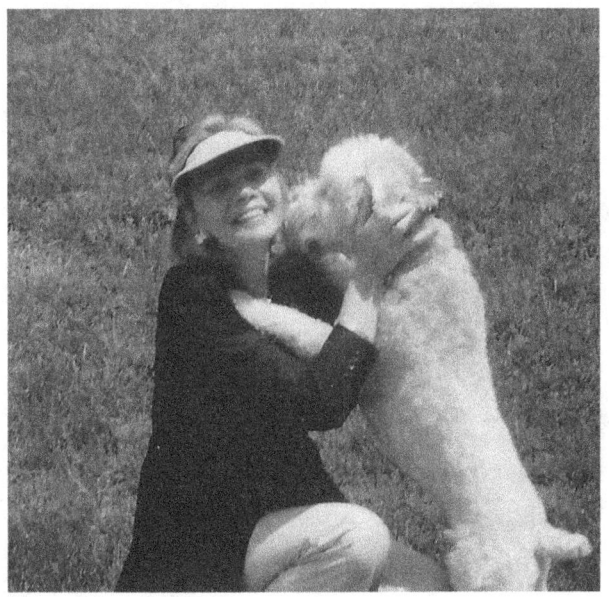

Phyllis—Stage 1

Phyllis was in the mild stage, I would guess, for three to four years. She could still drive to familiar places, but once, going from Washington, DC, to Connecticut, she circled the beltway around Washington (I-495) several times. Fortunately, she had a cell with my number programmed in, and I was able to direct her to the road to Baltimore and beyond. Her cell phone capability around that time (2004) was limited to calling only her siblings and my home and cell numbers. At that stage, Phyllis was still manageable, but remembering numbers, names, and places, being able to shop, and preparing meals were becoming increasingly difficult and unlikely.

In another instance, I put her on a plane to Cincinnati to visit her three siblings. Her brother was supposed to meet the flight, but he was late (obviously it is dangerous to be late when meeting a patient with Alzheimer's disease). She wandered around aimlessly and finally boarded an airport tram that was taking passengers from gate to gate. She thought the "train" was going into the city. She apparently got off at one gate, was confused, and after not reaching me on her cell, called my brother in Mexico. He, in turn, called Phyllis's sister Natalie in Cincinnati.

Nat later said, "If you want to get something done, send a woman." She called Phyllis and had her describe where she was as best she could. Nat said, "Stay right there," and she relayed her location to her brother, and he finally found Phyllis. The whole process took about two hours, but Phyllis seemed unperturbed and happy to see her brother. Scary!

Respite

Early on I sought out "respite time" (from nine o'clock until noon on Mondays through Fridays) at the local Alzheimer's disease center in Vero Beach. It was a godsend. For three hours, they would do simple crafts, sing songs, and socialize to a limited extent, which freed one up to do errands and write. On the days I dropped her off, they would keep her amused with group activities until noon. That went on for about three years until her motor skills and inability to socialize with others made attendance impossible.

The Alzheimer's disease center also provided a training session for caregivers. They simulated an Alzheimer's disease patient's environment and perception. My fingers were taped to show the awkwardness of Alzheimer's disease. An uncomfortable impediment was placed in each shoe to show transference problems. The room was almost completely dark except for one light. Blaring music was playing, and I was instructed to complete six simple tasks, including folding towels, filling a glass of water, and finding specific objects. The disorienting experience was shocking, and it was interesting that both the fire and police departments had to go through the same training procedure to increase their understanding of dementia victims.

When the time came, the Alzheimer's disease center provided information on various assisted living facilities, which I had just begun to consider.

Tip: Determine if there is an Alzheimer's office or facility in your community or other services that can provide "respite" or relief for you for a few hours. This limited time will provide you with free time and a chance to handle some of your own needs. Recharging your batteries is critical to the caregiver's well-being! Sometimes, nursing homes will board the care receiver so the caregiver can respite for a week or even a month.

Toward the end of what I assumed to be the early stage, we could still go out for dinner and talk, although at times, a conversation would be circular and eventually consisted mainly of non sequiturs. Still, she enjoyed talking and looking at the people. I am a typical type A male, and patience was not one of my virtues, but I had to learn it pretty quickly as Phyllis became more and more dependent on me.

The Alzheimer's Association gave me a card with the major dos and don'ts on it when dealing with an Alzheimer's victim, which was most helpful.

Tip: I would read this list ASAP (See list "The Ten Nevers").

One of the hardest things I had to learn on the list was never to argue. If she won the argument, I would lose. If I won the argument, she wouldn't remember—and I'd still lose. In any case, argument and criticism would only heighten agitation.

It was clear we were both undergoing behavior changes—hers because of the disease and mine due to the voluntary and involuntary requirements to accommodate her changing personality and needs.

Notes

The Ten Nevers

These are the ten "Nevers" the Alzheimer's Association provided me. Once your loved one is starting to show signs of forgetfulness or disorientation or other symptoms of mid-stage Alzheimer's, it would be good to employ these suggestions as appropriate:

<u>Never argue</u>. There is no percentage in this. You really can't win, but you can agitate the patient.

<u>Never reason</u>. But try to redirect the conversation.

<u>Never shame</u>. But try to distract the person's inappropriate words or actions.

<u>Never lecture</u>. You have to remember the Alzheimer's patient doesn't see logic or behavior in a cogent way.

<u>Never say</u>, "Remember when?" (She probably doesn't). Reminisce. To refer to something in the past, it would be better to reminisce than to put her on the spot. In fact, avoiding questions that can be confusing and frustrating to the care receiver is recommended.

<u>Never say</u>, "I already told you." This is very difficult for the caregiver, particularly in the early stages. I can remember Phyllis asking me where we were going four or five times in a five-minute ride. Frankly, that was the beginning of my lessons in patience, the need for which increased geometrically over time.

<u>Never say</u>, "You can't." Encourage them to do what they can unless it's destructive, then redirect.

<u>Never command</u>. Ask. Don't say, "Give me the pencil." Say, "Will you please give me the pencil?"

<u>Never condescend</u>. Encourage and praise. This is difficult to do, especially with childlike behavior, but you must imprint on your own mind that you are dealing with a different person because their brain does not function in logical, cogent ways as it once did.

<u>Never force</u>. Reinforce. For example, don't say, "Get in the car." Instead reinforce. I would say, "Come on, sweetie. Let's get in the car, and we will go for a fun ride."

Notes

Driving

The largest and most bitter issue between us was the car. After a couple of minor accidents, it was clear that Phyllis could no longer drive. This is a real-life change for both the caregiver and the receiver as, obviously, driving is a major source of an individual's independence. I asked our doctor to "prescribe" a driving test for Phyllis. This gave me a scapegoat and someone to blame for "taking" her car away.

> *Tip: When that terrible time comes and you have to take your loved one's driving ability away, I strongly suggest finding a scapegoat, preferably not a family member, but someone who will be perceived in an official capacity. If not, a lot of the anger and bitterness resulting from the driving restriction will be directed at you. And don't wait!*

In my case, Phyllis was more attached to driving her car than most people. Over the years, she would think nothing of jumping (alone) into her car and driving from Connecticut to see her mother in Cincinnati or Cape Coral, Florida. She would turn on talk radio, feel comfortably insulated, and drive for eight or ten hours. I knew what not driving and losing her car would mean to her.

The prescribed "driving test" was not in a car or on the road. It was in the laboratory setting where Phyllis had to identify street signs and use a simulator to test her reflexes to brake at a red light and put on the gas on the green light.

She also had to complete a mini memory test, which she had been doing in the neurologist's office over the previous two years with declining results. It asks such questions as:

- What is your name?
- Where do you live (county, state, town)?
- When were you born?
- Who is the president of the United States?
- Who was president before him?
- Remember three objects and tell them later (five minutes).
- Draw a clock face showing ten o'clock.
- Copy a geometrical figure.
- Where are you now?
- How would you drive home?

The test monitors cognitive ability over time, and it identifies specific weakness such as spatial relations (i.e., the geometry task).

At the outset of her Alzheimer's, Phyllis could answer about 90 percent of the thirty questions correctly. Therefore, it was a shock to see her fail to correctly answer "What city do you live in?" "Who is the president of the United States?" "What state do you live in?" Her scores would decline until, finally, she got to the point where she could only recall her first name.

After about an hour, the driving tester took me aside and asked, "You don't expect her to pass this test and continue driving, do you?"

"No," I said. "I really wanted independent confirmation that she shouldn't drive."

"Well, you will certainly have that," said the tester. "Her reflexes are only about 22 percent of normal, and she can only identify two out of the twelve road signs (stop and slow). She has no recognition of railroad crossings and other hazards."

At the conclusion of the test, the tester informed Phyllis that she could no longer drive. Her status as such would be forwarded to the state highway patrol and the local police department.

As we drove home, Phyllis was as mad as a hornet. "That was the stupidest woman. She should've known I was tired, and you shouldn't have brought me!"

She finally begrudgingly accepted the fact that her no-driving status was official. I felt very pleased that I had not tried to take the keys away from her myself and had used the doctor and the state testing center as the targets for her anger. She still harbored a bit of anger toward me for even driving her to the test site, but for the most part, I was off the hook.

In addition to Phyllis losing a huge amount of her independence, I also had to give up a chunk of my own. I became the person who did the grocery shopping, picked up the dry cleaning, chauffeured Phyllis to her doctors and dentists and hair appointments, cooked our meals, and cleaned up afterward. In other words, I was both husband and wife, but there was a lot more to come.

Tip: The Mini Mental State Exam (MMSE) is good to use as a gauge of memory decline, and you can conduct it yourself (http://www.Dementia.com).

Notes

Caregivers

After interviewing several caregiver agencies, I started with the caregiver coming for only three hours per day and not live-in help. Although this left me with considerable work still for Phyllis and myself, it was a nice respite. Added to the three hours at the Alzheimer center, it virtually gave me six hours alone to do things such as having lunch with friends, going to my own appointments, paying bills, and occasionally playing a round of golf.

Every weekday morning, I would make Phyllis a protein shake with egg and then drive her to the Alzheimer center for her three-hour social time. On Fridays, there was a piano player they all loved. It was amazing to me to see twenty or more Alzheimer's disease victims sitting in a circle, many of whom could not tell you where they lived or even their spouse's name, but they were able to remember the golden oldies word for word. A favorite was "Old MacDonald Had a Farm."

Incidentally, music is excellent for Alzheimer's victims because in order to "hear" the notes, their brains have to encode the sound waves into notes and then decode the notes in order to reach the synapses of the brain. Music exercises the brain just as you would exercise an atrophied muscle. Not surprisingly, new studies have shown that music can dramatically improve the mood of Alzheimer's disease patients and is probably better than conventional drugs in slowing the disease's progression.

Tip: If you can, provide the care receiver with music. When Phyllis was in nursing homes, I would set up an old cell phone with Pandora and a Bluetooth speaker that played continuous and relatively calm music. The nurses would turn it off at night, and I would turn it on the next day.

At noon, the caregiver would pick up Phyllis at the Alzheimer's disease center and take her off for lunch and then for grocery shopping, hair, or nails. Usually I would take her to any doctor's appointment so I could communicate with the doctor.

However, for certain appointments, such as a dentist, I would let the caregiver take her and wait for her in the waiting room. Also, I tried to delegate certain errands to the caregiver such as the dry cleaner, hairdresser, and clothes shopping for Phyllis. By that time, she had moved away from her elegant clothes to simpler fare. Usually she would wear elastic, warm-up pants for quick-changing purposes with a blouse or simple shirt. A very glamorous addition to her wardrobe was Depends (diapers), which eventually became a round-the-clock staple.

Tip: Screen agencies and the caregivers they provide. And for God's sake, make sure they can drive and have a car.

After a couple of months of this three-hour routine, I moved to an eight-hour session—for the caregiver. This would give me almost half a day on my own and would carry Phyllis through dinner. As an aside, it was not cheap—eight hours a day runs about $160, and on a six-day basis amounts to $960 per week. On Sundays, I would take Phyllis to church, lunch, and then home for a kid's movie or a football game on TV.

Fortunately, my long-term-care insurance covered this after a ninety-day exclusion period. (This is not to be confused with the ninety-day exclusion period you have to face when you move your loved one into a facility such as a hospital or nursing home.)

As Phyllis's life slipped into an abyss, I eventually made a deal with the caregiver agency to have one of our favorite caregivers come to live in but not charge me for more than half a day. By mounting a video camera in the caregiver's room, and focused on Phyllis, she was able to sleep through the night. Otherwise, the caregiver would have to stay awake in the room with the patient for the entire night. And that, my friends, would be $480 per day, which is prohibitive for most people ($14,400 per month) and only partially covered by my fairly liberal long-term-care policy.

Of course, the caregiver or I would have to check Phyllis once or twice during the night to see if she needed changing.

Tip: If your loved one is going to sleep alone, a video baby monitor is recommended—and perhaps an alarm that sounds whenever she gets out of bed. This should be checked with local authorities as legal policies on these suggestions vary by state and community.

This program worked for a while, but things became more complicated when Phyllis could no longer dress herself in the morning. She resisted my help. She became incontinent and was at risk of wandering, which meant she had to be under supervision every waking moment. We live in a gated community, so I instructed the guards—if

Phyllis

they saw my wife walking alone or trying to leave the community on her own—to quickly call me and do what they could to prevent her from departing the premises.

Notes

Full-Time Home Care

At one point, I was having a caregiver coming into the house for eight hours a day, which was very helpful since the increasing care required was becoming more burdensome, particularly as we got into problems of dressing, bathrooming, and hygiene. Added to this were the continuing chores of doing the shopping, dry cleaning, preparing meals, washing up, dressing, medicating and putting Phyllis to bed—plus changing her diapers during the night, showers in the morning, dressing her, giving her breakfast, and getting her to the Alzheimer's disease center by nine. Besides this daily routine, I had to frequently take Phyllis to various doctors, dentists, hair appointments, and the nail salon. It was our objective to keep Phyllis looking beautifully well-groomed as she had been over the years.

The 36-Hour Day, a very popular information book on Alzheimer's, describes exactly what each day feels like for the family or caregiver.

Tip: I recommend reading The 36-Hour Day. While my book is a personal adventure, The 36-Hour Day is more of a comprehensive textbook or guide.

It has been stated that:

- Forty-eight percent of caregivers die before their care receivers.
- Providing intensive caregiving, particularly of a loved one, can deduct at least four years from your normal life expectancy.

I don't know how they conducted the research that came up with these two factors, but after several years of caregiving, I sometimes felt they underestimated the "drag" on the caregiver's life. It becomes a full-time job—and then some.

Tip: At the moderate stage, the Alzheimer's center also supplied Phyllis with a GPS tracking bracelet. I recommend using this bracelet as soon as practical—plus a medical ID bracelet—hopefully before the moderate stage, especially if the patient can still leave wherever she is living. This became less critical in a memory care facility since they are almost universally "locked down."

Notes

Nursing Home Types

After reading up on the subject and visiting various types of nursing homes, the following alternatives were available in my area. . They generally give a wide definition of nursing homes as "any facility you can board and receive some level of care you cannot provide for yourself."

Assisted Living Facilities

These homes are targeted for those individuals who have certain problems and cannot live totally independently. Many assisted living facilities have separate suites or apartments that provide attractive living quarters, including bathrooms and, in some cases, sitting rooms. These facilities are generalized and accept people with various conditions that are not solely oriented to cognitive and dementia problems. In my experience, they provide three meals a day, entertainment, limited chair exercises, occasional shopping or theater trips, and other events to occupy the residents. Residents generally eat in a common dining room that provides some level of socialization. There are also libraries, television sets, and beauty salons available, and most assisted living facilities are prepared to provide support services. In Phyllis's case, those included changing, dressing, bathing, bathrooming, and, most important, dispensing medication. Pricing is all over the lot, but $4,000–$10,000 per month seems to be the range in Florida. In the Northeast, it can be as much as 50 percent higher.

Note: rates generally have exceeded "cost of living" annual increases.

Memory Care

Memory care units are usually the last step for Alzheimer's disease patients. Some assisted living facilities also have separate memory care units that are locked up at entry and provide comfortable non-hospital settings such as suites and apartments and mostly consist of dementia patients who are in danger of wandering. As more care is required, fees may be 10–15 percent higher than assisted living facilities.

Skilled Nursing

Patients who are even more debilitated may need round-the-clock nursing and have to "graduate" to a skilled nursing facility. A memory care unit in some cases can also provide the equivalent of skilled nursing with a further monthly upcharge.

Continuing Care Retirement Communities

I also recommend exploring one-stop shopping as in the case of continuing care retirement communities which I describe in some detail below.

To avoid some of the pitfalls I fell into involving many different moves for Phyllis—a total of eleven in-and-out moves—plus all the administrative paperwork that piles up—for peace of mind you may want to consider a Continuing Care Retirement Community. Doing this will require some foresight and planning since you pretty much have to enter the facility while you are in good health.

Most continuing care retirement communities have apartments or cottages for independent living, assisted living when individuals can no longer totally take care of themselves, and skilled nursing when even more care is required than assisted living. In this manner, it provides a sort of rest-of-life solution. Most continuing care retirement communities such as the largest, which is ACTS, will require an entry fee ("buy-in") that can run from $60,000–$280,000 for a one-bedroom unit, depending on geography and the type of apartment you require, plus a monthly fee (i.e., $2,000–3,000 per month) to cover maintenance, dining, and other services. If you or your partner are already diagnosed with Alzheimer's, I'm not sure you would pass the "nurse's entry exam." However, if one of you is in the very early stages and self-sufficient, they may allow you to qualify for independent living. Obviously, the cost of assisted living and skilled nursing is considerably greater than independent living.

Therefore, they want to make sure that you do not sign up and require advanced care the next day. The entry fee is partially tax-deductible, up to 40 percent, because it is, in effect, prepaying for future medical services according to the IRS. Part of your monthly fee is also deductible, but usually not more than 10 percent, and the balance is perceived as feeding and housing. The entry fees can also be reduced by about 30 percent if you have existing long-term-care policies. As stated, the monthly fee might also carry a slight discount of about 10 percent as the burden of your advanced care can be reduced by long-term-care claims reimbursements.

If you and your partner are in reasonable health, I suggest looking into the CCRC solution. The CCRC choice is much like an insurance policy in that it stabilizes your future medical costs and situates you and your spouse in the same overall facility for your lifetimes.

To summarize, the advantages of the CCRC:

- You will receive excellent medical healthcare for the rest of your life.
- You will remain in the same community as your partner/spouse even if you are in different locations according to your health needs.
- Your kids and family will be assured that the financial burden of old age will not fall on them.
- Your entry fee can be returned in part if you leave the facility within four years. Generally, the returned fee is reduced by 25 percent for each of the first four years.
- You (and your spouse) will receive meals, cleaning, maintenance, and care for life.
- You will have a number of group activities, exercise, games, and hopefully friends to keep you mentally alert and physically fit.
- Your monthly costs will be considerably lower than facilities that do not have continuing care.

These are today's costs* for the different facilities in Florida (estimated 2017 rates):

- Regular ALF: $5–12K/month
- Skilled nursing: $10–15K/month
- CCRC: $2–4K/month
- In home 24/7 caregiver: $14–15K/month

*Depending on geography

Of course, the one-time entry fees are considerably higher for the CCRC than the community fee in nursing homes, but they frequently can be offset by the sale of your current home, and once paid, you only have to deal with the monthly fee. In some cases, part of the down payment for CCRCs can be returned when you leave.

Looking back on what I coulda, woulda, shoulda done, at the earliest sign of Phyllis's memory loss—and before she was diagnosed with Alzheimer's disease—would have been signing up for a CCRC. It would have saved a lot of emotional Sturm und Drang—not to speak of considerable savings over the years she was afflicted. We could have "bought in" to a condo or cottage. Once Phyllis's condition worsened, she could move to advanced care in the same facility

The assisted living facilities that told me she could be there for life were totally inaccurate. She was evicted from three facilities. As mentioned, the first said, "Of course she can stay with a private nurse 24/7." The second said, "She can't return unless she is ambulatory." The third said, "Her fits are too loud and disturbing."

Example: $100,000 Entry Fee
(Florida Experience)

		CCRC	Nursing Home
Phase I	1-Bdrm Apt/ Condo	$2,500/mo.	$4,000–5,000/mo.
Phase II	Assisted Living	$2,500/mo.	$6,000–8,000/mo.
Phase III	Skilled Nursing	$2,500/mo.	$10,000–14,000/mo.

Note: The entry fee is often positioned as a "buy-in" fee, but in reality, it is a payment for an "insurance policy" that will cover your future care. In most cases, you are not "purchasing the unit," and it reverts back to the facility when you and your spouse move on to the next stage.

Note: In other continuing care retirement communities, you buy your cottage or condo, and when you vacate, you must sell it back to the facility for 90 percent of your original purchase price. You can assume they will sell it to another potential resident for much more than you paid—and certainly a great deal more than your return of 90 percent. If one of you does not qualify as "healthy" and needs extra care, they will revert to market price for a nursing home (as shown in the table above).

CCRC is a pretty good deal because initially you can live in a cottage or apartment/condo, possibly for years. Then, if you or your spouse need more care, they can move out independently to assisted or memory care while you remain in your "home."

What happens if, after five years of living in your apartment with your spouse, you are no longer able to care for yourself? You are moved to the "assisted living" section within the complex at no increase in monthly charges of say $3,000 per month. If your situation worsens in a couple of years, and you cannot do the basics for yourself (transportation, walking, bathrooming, grooming, hygiene, dressing), you will be moved to assisted living or skilled nursing (which provides extensive care in more of a hospital setting) with no increase in your monthly fee in Acts' communities, except for possible cost of living increase of 3 percent per year, which is also the case if you remained in independent care.

Note: A long-term-care policy could reduce the entry fee 25–30 percent and the monthly rate by 10 percent. However, if one of you is self-sufficient, they can remain in the apartment/cottage at no increased cost. This should be negotiated up front!

This is a good program for controlling your later-in-life health expenses since assisted living facilities can run $5,000–$8,000 per month (at current prices), and round-the-clock skilled nursing can run considerably more.

Maintenance fees* usually include:

- at least thirty meals per month
- fitness activities
- educational classes
- "Samaritan fund" financial safety net to safeguard you financially
- tax benefits and deductions of 39–41 percent of entry fees considered by the IRS as prepaid deductible medical expenses
- partial write-off of monthly fee.

At the same time, if you have long-term care, your admission fees could be reduced by 25–30 percent and monthly charges by 10 percent. This is due to the fact that long-term-care claims would offset at least a part of future care needs and costs.

* Fees may vary widely based on geography and the quality of the facility.

Notes

Long-Term Care

While having a long-term-care policy for Phyllis was helpful for me and furnished up to $8,000 per month for six years, long-term-care insurance policies may be in some jeopardy. Insurance companies have actually misforecasted three critical areas:

- overestimated the number of policies that would be canceled without claims.
- the interest returns that could be earned on investment of premiums (3 percent versus 7 percent forecasted)
- the life expectancy of a sixty-five-year-old male, which jumped from 18.1 years in 1990 to 21.7 in 2015.

This has created a significant financial drain on insurance companies such as Penn Treaty, which has 79,000 policyholders, according to the *Wall Street Journal,* for a projected liability of $4 billion in future claims compared to their $600 million in assets. I would imagine similar situations exist with major insurance companies; consequently, premiums will become larger, and coverage will become smaller. This is symbolic of some basic facts that impact both the medical and the insurance business; actuaries, years ago, did not project the graying of America and the medical and care costs of the millions of aged who will have to be warehoused in some manner of institution in the future.

Fortunately, for the very poor, Medicaid covers a major part if not all of institutionalization, but for the rest of Americans, care of elders does and will present major financial liabilities going forward. In the other event of an insurance company failure, the industry is looking into assessments for other insurance companies to make up the shortfalls. However, in the long run, this would simply exacerbate the financial problems facing the long-term-care insurance industry.

Tip: If you're in the market for long-term-care insurance, check into the financial stability of the offering companies and determine if there is any fine print concerning the consequences of the company's inability to pay future claims, particularly for Alzheimer's disease and cancer.

Daily Long-Term Care Benefits (My Experience)

Year	$ With Inflation Rider (5% simple)	$ Without
1	160	160
5	200	160
10	240	160
12	256	160
Current Monthly Max (2017)	7,670	4,800

As you can see, twelve years ago, $4,800/month might have offset a major portion, if not all, of your initial costs, but twelve years later, they cover only a small fraction of your daily coverage since assisted living facilities cost between $5,000 and $14,000/month and vary regionally. Therefore, I recommend the inflation rider if you are considering these policies.

Tip: If you do get a long-term-care policy, opt for the annual cost increase rider to more or less keep up with inflation (see table above).

Although preplanning by purchasing a long-term-care policy or signing up for a CCRC is not acted upon—most people in good health do not foresee the possible (and most likely) need for considerable health care down the road—up to 26 percent of Medicaid/Medicare, and up to 80 percent of total medicine, is spent on the last five years of people's lives. Without protective measures, your golden years may be tarnished.

Notes

Moderate Stage 2

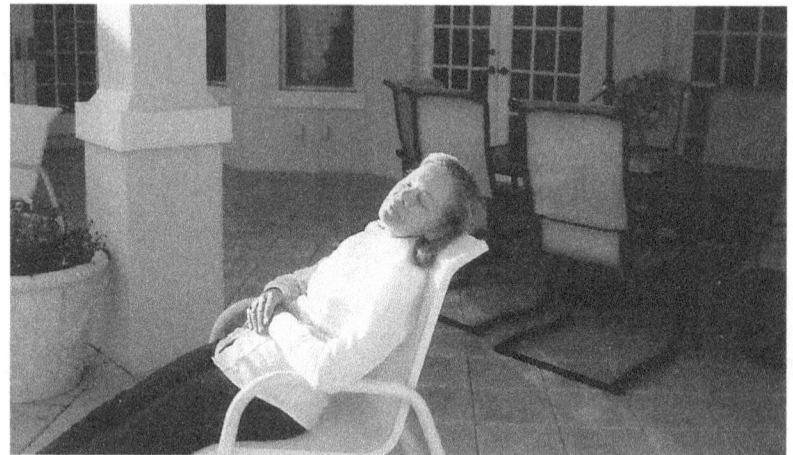

Phyllis—Stage 2

Although the lines between the stages in Alzheimer's disease are blurred and the sequence of behavior changes varies between individuals, I realized Phyllis was losing more and more of her life each day. She could still walk alone, but she could no longer dress herself appropriately, shower, brush her teeth, and "bathroom" herself (an awkward but descriptive verb).

As conversation was limited, we would watch a lot of TV in the evenings. Nature shows, sports, and quiz shows were the best since she was completely lost on any plotted programs. After many months of live-in caregiving and scouting out all the assisted living facilities in the area, we decided to move her to what unfortunately turned out to be the first of her several institutional experiences.

Tip: From a tour and the appearances of the facility, it is hard to determine which assisted living facility will best suit the Alzheimer's disease patient. Use this following checklist before committing to any facility, including assisted living facility, memory care, skilled nursing, or continuing care retirement communities.

1. Obviously, you and/or a family member should take a tour of the various facilities available to you in the community where you would want to live.
2. What are your observations and feelings about the environment, layout, and interior decorating?
3. How efficient does the facility appear?
4. How does the motivation of the staff seem—particularly their attitudes toward the residents?

5. What exercise, activities, and events do they have for the residents in a typical month.
6. What will your monthly fee include? What percentage increases have occurred in those fees over the past three to five years? If they are running more than three, you have to at least question in your own mind how efficient they are and how financially sound the organization is.
7. What transportation do they provide to doctors' appointments, shopping, and entertainment?
8. What is the occupancy rate? If it is much under 80 percent, it raises concerns about financial stability.
9. Will they share their recent audited financial statements with you or your designated representative (CPA, eldercare lawyer, or accountant)? Can they review your contract?
10. Are all the proper licenses in effect and on display?
11. In the case of continuing care retirement communities, you should be clear about the services they provide in their continuing care. Also, review their skilled nursing and other living facilities.

With my growing responsibilities for the household and a lot of things Phyllis had normally handled before Alzheimer's disease, I realized we had left the early phase of the disease and had to consider one of the different types of homes for her.

Even though I checked out all the neighboring assisted living facilities, I felt it was still too early to expel Phyllis from the house even though wandering was still a potential problem.

Running through my mind was Orson Bean's quip: "I live in a gated community, but my wife still gets out."

Early in the game, as suggested, you should get a medical alert bracelet (available at most chain pharmacies) for your care receiver. Even though the silver bracelet said "Alzheimer's" on the back, Phyllis liked it, probably couldn't read the disease, and would proudly show it to friends.

Remote Family and Friends

According to several of the Alzheimer's disease books I read, the challenge of "remote relations or friends" seems to arise as a serious concern. As I was trying to do my best for Phyllis, I greatly underestimated the pressure from family "help" and second-guessing.

Most books mention that remote family, when the assisted living facility subject comes up, feel the caregiver is moving the loved one out of the home too soon.

"But she is so happy at home." "She doesn't know anyone in the facility." "When we visit, we can all be under the same roof." "She will be close to her familiar belongings."

The books generally go on to say your own sense of abandoning her, plus the guilt trip provided by the "remotes," the caregiver tends to "institutionalize" the care receiver much later than they should for the optimal care of both the Alzheimer's disease-afflicted person and the caregiver.

"Besides," the remote relative states, "you have Annie from the agency in for five hours a day, five days a week. Before you move Phyllis, just extend the hours a bit, and you will have more time for yourself." Easy for them to say as they visit and then go home.

At first, it seemed like a reasonable argument. I kept Phyllis at home for a few more months—after her first two negative experiences in nursing homes—even though she was becoming less and less manageable and required more and more care. Facing up to the facts, despite the family, I continued my survey of memory facilities with the thought that Phyllis would need more care than I could provide—even with a full-time professional caregiver.

In a matter of months, if not weeks, I had been told to keep Phyllis safe at home, I had to install alarms on all the doors and bed, highly placed locks for the doors (preferably combination), grips for the showers and toilets, and cushioned carpets for the hallways. Sooner or later, Alzheimer's patients become fall risks. All dangerous and precious objects should be hidden, and the knives should be removed from the kitchen drawers and put in high and inaccessible places. Ideally, I was told, the pool should be enclosed with a fence to prevent her from wandering into it. As I figured, Phyllis would be with me for just a short time more. I procrastinated on the structural changes and installing the suggested hardware additions to the bathrooms.

After fifty years of sharing a bed with my wife, she became incontinent. Even with the diapers and rubber sheets, our first "separation" occurred when I moved her over to the spare bedroom. At that point, Phyllis started to pace the house and would hide things under her mattress. As is typical with Alzheimer's, Phyllis also started "sundowners," which are usually afternoon times of agitation, anger, and even sometimes hitting. Initially, these sundowners took me by surprise—even though I was warned by my reading. I would see a complete transformation of my well-tempered wife. She would switch into an anger-filled Jekyll and Hyde mode for an hour or more. That was where patience really came to the fore. A woman who told you minutes before that she loved you "more than anything in the world" would suddenly turn on you, calling you "disgusting," insulting anyone else in the room sometimes with language I had never heard from her mouth. The medical profession still cannot identify the cause of these chemical changes.

You cannot talk them down from the sundowners! You cannot aggressively react to the attacks on yourself. You can try to distract with some desired object or discussion of a family member. Generally, all you can do is take it on the chin and try to prevent her from hurting someone when she tries to strike them, while she contorts her face like some scene from *The Exorcist*, and directs hateful phrases at everyone.

Obviously, anger and logic have no place in the discussion and argument should never be engaged. It was clear to me that the person I had known and loved all these years was no longer present during these sieges. I was thankful that I had read so much about the disease and realized, although it was atypical for her personality, it was not unusual for Alzheimer's disease patients. However, at that juncture, I began to realize we were either at the beginning of stage 3 or the end of stage 2. There are no firm boundaries or demarcations that definitively define the stages of Alzheimer's.

Many books I've read and movies I have seen (e.g., *Still Alice, Glen Campbell*) seem to depict early Alzheimer's disease and genuinely describe the disease up to a point, but they erroneously leave us with a false sense of hope with couples walking hand in hand toward the setting sun while dramatic music and the credits start to roll.

I hope to give you a clearer, but greater insight into the late phase and end-of-life expectations and alternatives. Unless they come up with a miraculous cure for this disease in the next few years, there are really no reprieves for the patient's life and the toll on his or her family as described within. However, for the loving caregiver, if there are any positives to come out of this dreadful disease, you quickly learn a lot about yourself and how you cope throughout this protracted ordeal and the incredible amount of patience required. You may also learn who your real friends are and perhaps gain a greater understanding of what matters in your life plus a perspective on your own prevailing values and how quickly you have to shift gears just to deal with each day and the surprises it can bring.

Just as AA stipulates, your first step should be to admit there is a power greater than yourself. This will be helpful during the ordeal to come—whether you are care receiver or caregiver. This power should not be used for taking out your rage and blame; instead use it as a companion you seek out for consultation, guidance, feedback, and prayer.

Advanced Stage 3

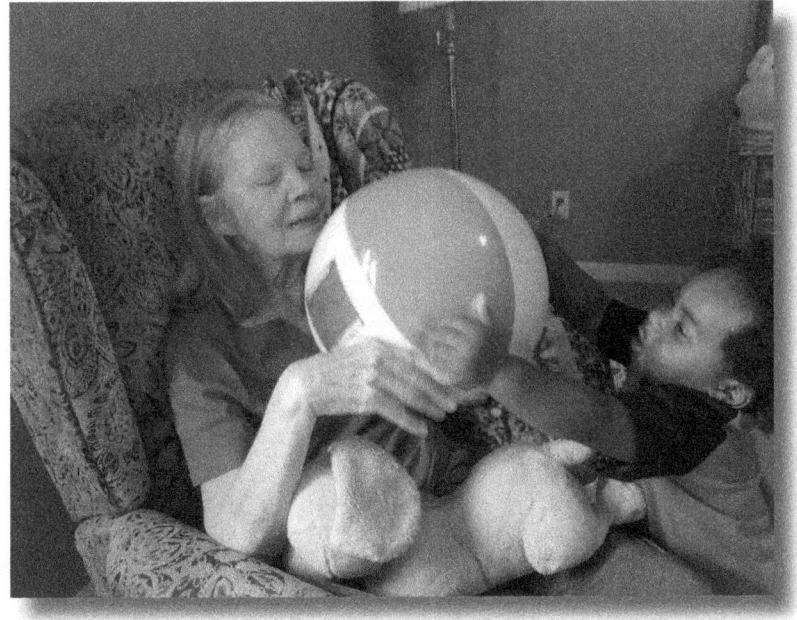

Phyllis—Stage 3

Alzheimer's disease victims often say, "I want to go home." This is not a location or geographic request. It is a cry out for a return to the familiar—childhood, parents, their former cogent life, a touchstone to reality—when things were better.

"Where are Mom and Dad?" Phyllis frequently asked.

It was also a request to return to security, to the familiar, to ask why she was "lost." These pleas were emotionally upsetting and wrenching for me, but I was told I had to remember it was the disease talking.

Along with mood changes, sundowners become prevalent in the majority of Alzheimer's disease victims in late stage 2 or early 3. These usually occur later in the afternoon and evening when depression may prevail. The darkness is coming. I've lost another day. There appears to be no hope!" (Non-Alzheimer's disease victims tend to call this the cocktail hour.)

There is no set way to deal with sundowning. Fatigue may be a factor, and a daily nap after lunch may help. (Phyllis could be quite active, pacing the room, calling ugly names, hiding car keys or pieces of mail under her mattress. In later stage 3, she would even hit people who were trying to calm her.)

After a while, Phyllis's sundowners changed to fits of crying, sobbing, and screaming, obviously worse than "normal" sundowners. Our gerontologist diagnosed this as pseudobulbar affect (PBA), which added more costly medication to the list. This partially reduced the PBA, but she was still considered disruptive to the nursing home and, as we found out, apparently to all care facilities.

It was incredibly painful to see anyone so distraught, much less my beloved wife of over fifty years. Pseudobulbar affect is not necessarily a symptom of Alzheimer's disease, nor is Parkinson's, but it often accompanies dementia cases.

When I would visit Phyllis at the assisted living facility, she frequently would smile, cling to my arm, and say, "Hello, sweetie. I love you more than anything." On these occasions, I frequently felt she thought I had come to spring her from the locked-down facility and take her "home." She was always disappointed! On other occasions, and only a few seconds after she grabbed my arm and called me "sweetie," her face, again, would do a Jekyll and Hyde and contort like the girl in *The Exorcist* and say, "I hate you. you are disgusting. I hate everyone!" It was so contrary to her personality. I was convinced it was the disease and unimaginable frustration.

As you might imagine, the uncontrollable sobbing, keening, and screaming—unlike any human distress I ever heard, even in horror movies—was totally unnerving for all of us. Several Alzheimer's disease books and sources claimed she was not as upset as her behavior appeared, which I tried to believe, especially when she would forget her hysterics minutes later.

However, her distress and sadness were so real. The outbreaks may not have stayed with her, but they certainly haunted me! It continued to unnerve me and intensify my sense of guilt. I felt somehow—in some way—I should have prevented such tragic circumstances. The hysterical outbreaks were much worse than the sundowners. In Phyllis's case, they necessitated a private room because the screaming sessions would greatly disturb any roommate.

Tip: As your loved one has sundowners or sinks into depression, try to be aware of certain triggers. For example, when Phyllis's sister came to see her, Phyllis went into immediate paroxysms of unabated sobbing. The sight of her sister brought back her youth, her parents, her early life on the farm, and some realization of her current state. A call from her brother George resulted in the same effect, particularly when he used his childhood name of "Georgie." Some triggers may be simply a chemical change or misalignment of the synapses in her brain—and may not be for any other reasons—but alertness to sensory triggers may help you eliminate, understand, or at least reduce the outbreaks.

Notes

Finances

As the quality of my own life was declining rapidly, I made that first choice for a nursing home. Fortunately, I had purchased a long-term-care insurance policy for both of us back in 2002, which defrayed a large percentage of legitimate professional care in either the home or in a licensed institution, including assisted living facilities, nursing homes, and memory care units.

Be aware of frequent price increases as demand and operating costs increase and anticipate a lag in your cash flow since insurance companies take forty to sixty days to pay for each completed month after the fact. Your lag time can also be increased if the administrator in your facility does not submit the claims exactly as required by the insurance company. I had a problem with this in four institutions I used; submissions can be sloppy, and insurance companies love the cash float of returning the claim if not properly presented. At one point in 2015, I was $90,000 behind in reimbursements. By the next year, I was $140,000 in the hole.

Also, be aware that most assisted living facilities have a nonreturnable "community cost" of $2,000–$3,000 initially. Compounding this, most insurance companies have a ninety-day "exclusion" period for institutional care, and this is over and above the ninety-day exclusion period for home care. So, if you add together the community cost, the first month in advance, the ninety-day exclusion, and the lag time in reimbursement, you can be looking at six months out of your pocket before you see a dime.

Once the system is "grooved," your cash flow will even out. There are, of course, other costs: supplies, medications, and most assisted living facilities require you furnish the room(s). Be ready to get into the furniture moving game.

Tip: If you don't have long-term-care insurance, get it as soon as possible for you and your spouse—the earlier age-wise, the better (and the cheaper). This should be done before there is any formal diagnosis of Alzheimer's; otherwise, the policy may be ineffective. Also, opt for the benefit inflation rider of at least 5 percent per year to increase your long-term-care coverage. Unfortunately, the increases are calculated on a simple interest basis, but nevertheless, they can provide an important offset to part or all of the increasing price of institutionalization.

Tip: If you have long-term insurance, make sure that clear requirements of the insurance company for the monthly claim reimbursement are provided to the assisted living facility. (They will still probably screw it up for a while.)

Note: If you set up a CCRC (as described) you may not need the long-term-care premiums year after year since your health care needs are covered by your monthly and entry fees. However, having long-term care may reduce your entry fee by 30 percent and your monthly payment by 10 percent, according to ACTS. You will have to do the math on this to determine if you are paying for double coverage.

In my recounting of Alzheimer's disease experiences, I may have had unusually bad experiences and overemphasized the financial impact, but added to the emotional stress I felt for my wife and over her care, it constituted a tremendous pressure upon me.

Fortunately, as in all of Florida, there were several assisted living facilities in Vero Beach. I toured them all and questioned their management and nursing staff. Each assured me that my wife would receive excellent care, safety, healthy meals, and be able to remain there the rest of her life. This did not turn out to be the case in any of the facilities we used, as I will explain.

Having "Mom at home" sounds great, especially to those who don't have to experience it. Even with the caregiver, I still had to be Mr. Mom. Although I only had to cover thirteen hours of the day, it was still affecting my life goals and, frankly, my happiness. The increasing sadness connected with Phyllis's disease, and living a life of service with very little enjoyment weighed heavily on me.

In many ways, it was great to have Phyllis at home. We had been companions for more than half a century, and she felt comfortable and safe in our king-sized bed. However, I still had to face the fact that, as things worsened, we both would be better off with her in a home.

At some point, you will have to realize that some friends will initially rally around you, but your social activities will decline considerably if your loved one is not able to participate in parties, group dinners, or other social functions. I was suddenly a lone, single man with a sick wife, and while our friends tried to include me in their parties, I would always throw off the dinner seating as the extra man. Another consideration is the wear and tear on the caregiver of a loved one. As you might imagine, I spent considerable time reading up on all aspects of the disease and the limited medications that do no more than possibly delay the decline. By the time I started looking for assisted living facilities, we needed round-the-clock caregiving at home. No matter how helpful one or more caregiver is, their around-the-clock presence limits your privacy and takes no prisoners when it comes to your wallet.

Tip: If the care receiver sleeps in a separate room from either you or a caregiver, a video baby monitor is a must. Also, you may avoid paying a caregiver for an all-night vigil since the monitor obviates the need for paying a caregiver while she is sleeping. This should be agreed to beforehand by the caregiver and/or her agency.

With this arrangement, I was able to reduce my daily home care bill from $450 per day to half. I used the round-the-clock in-home caregiver for eight months after my first two facilities' experience and before my second memory care facility. To recap our experiences:

Phyllis

Home I	Assisted Living Facility	5 months	Ejected because of fear of wandering, needed 24/7 nursing to stay (cost $22K/month).
Home II	Memory Care	4 months	Voluntarily left because of overmedication.
At Home	Home Care	8 months	Brought Phyllis home for the summer and through the Christmas holidays.

Home III	Memory Care	9 months	Until hospitalized for broken hip. Facility rejected return "if not ambulatory."
Home IV	Rehab	7 months	Ejected because of disruption to other patients due to periodic screaming (pseudobulbar affect).
Home V	Private Home	4 months	Until they called 911 for ER.
HH	Hospice House	3 days	Until death.

Notes

Financial Alternatives

While Phyllis was still attending respite care at the Alzheimer center from Monday through Friday, there was a meeting there for husbands of Alzheimer's disease victims every other Friday morning. The meetings were both depressing and enlightening. The men were mostly retired and in their eighties. None had any long-term-care insurance, and hearing their stories was almost heartbreaking. They all appeared to be beaten down by the consequences of being responsible for their wives, and in most cases, they didn't have the money for a home care or assisted living facilities. The images of these older men trying to deal with noncognitive and mostly incontinent women, changing them, dressing, driving, and dealing with their other physical problems—especially urinary tract infections which are so common with Alzheimer's disease—were almost impossible to imagine. Since paying for home care or even an assisted living facility was out of reach for most spouse caregivers, it was easy to see why arguably the caregiver loses four years of life expectancy and 48 percent die before their care receivers. In the case of these octogenarians, I bet the numbers were even higher. What happens when the caregiver dies first? Do the kids step in?

At these support group meetings, guest speakers would cover useful subjects and try to market assisted living facilities and other services. At one session, our guest was an "eldercare" lawyer who made some interesting suggestions and recommendations on legal and financial matters:

Using Medicaid

If you shifted your spouse's income and assets from her to you, you might have her qualify for Medicaid, but you would have to start the process three years ahead of the change. I rejected this out of hand since our joint assets would exceed the maximum allowed for Medicaid. However, if the assets were shifted to the patient's spouse or other family members, in theory Phyllis could drop below the poverty line and individually meet the low-asset requirements for Medicaid.

Because most of our assets were jointly held— our home, retirement portfolio, and some other investments—we would need to move around a lot of assets. Also, Phyllis had a few stocks and investments in her own name that would have to be sold or gifted. She also had a small IRA in her name, which again, would have to be liquidated. Obviously, a lot of work would have to be done to have a joint property ownership shifted to the caregiver or other family members. However, if it was done, Medicaid could kick in and cover a huge amount of increasing costs of Alzheimer's disease. I had not done that because, down deep, I felt it was a little shifty for us, but it was probably okay for the desperate. We also had long-term-care insurance, which in theory would cover a large percentage of our institutional costs. However, for some of the desperate caregiving men who saw no light at the end of the tunnel, the asset move was a considerable financial opportunity by going ahead and shifting assets and having Medicaid largely support their spouse's illness.

Tip: The IRS is aware of this practice and may do a three-year "look back" to see if you have a marked change in your assets or income. The greater the transfer of funds, the more scrutiny you can expect. Take care.

Reverse Mortgages

Another suggestion was the use of a reverse first mortgage. Many of these older people had considerable equity in their homes, which could be released by a reverse mortgage. For example, I actually used a reverse mortgage. My house's original cost was $750,000, and I took out a reverse mortgage for $400,000, about the extent of my equity interest, and the loan was contractually compounded at 5 percent per year. I assumed the market price increases on my house, plus entire property, my loan, would grow at a greater rate than the mortgage debt.

WITH the mortgage of $400,000 at 5 percent per annum versus the total house value growing at least 3 percent per annum, I assumed that I would never go underwater. In any case, if it did, the government via HUD would cover any loss when I sold, so I could not in theory "lose money" on the deal. Also, all the mortgage (P&I) payments were deferred until I sold or left the house, so I had no monthly mortgage payments. This seemed to be working well until we had the 2007 real estate crisis. In 2006, my house had been valued by Zillow at $1,250,000. By 2008, the same house value dropped to around $600,000 which was about equal to my reverse mortgage balance after ten years of compounding. At that point,

I really had no equity in the house. But if I sold my house for less than my outstanding balance on the reverse mortgage, the government would cover the difference, including a lot of the closing and brokerage costs.

Despite my bad luck and timing, reverse mortgages can be a viable way for homeowners over sixty-two to reduce their monthly expenses and also take out the lion's share of the equity in the house to help defray medical and other expenses. Plus, there is a guarantee that the owner(s) can never lose money on the eventual sale of their house. One of the drawbacks to reverse mortgages is that you cannot rent it out or transfer the house to your surviving children or even close friends. Any sale has to be an arm's-length deal, and you generally have a year to dispose of the house after you move.

For obvious reasons, the reverse mortgage should be at a fixed rate and not collectible until the house is resold or, at the latest, one year after the owner's departure. At that point, the "bank" would not be able to collect more than the amount of the sale, so there would be no further indebtedness on the part of the homeowner. Any remaining equity in the house would revert to the homeowner; however, the compounding of the annual interest rate would probably eat up most of this equity, and in many cases, it will exceed it.

Tip: With a reverse mortgage, part of the annual interest might be tax-deductible as mortgage interest. You may want to discuss this with your tax advisor because reverse mortgage interest write-offs can be treated differently by certain states.

Notes

Nursing Home I

After serious reconnoitering of the various assisted living facilities in the area (fortunately, the long-term-care policy made most of the facilities affordable), I selected the best, which had a private suite with a bath and a back door that led to a patio with a large walled-in garden area.

Upon paying my "community fee" (a nonrefundable placement fee—$2,500 in my case) we started the moving process: bed, couch, recliner, bureau, wall art, family pictures, name-tagged clothing, and towels. After the kids and I finished decorating the suite, it was a pretty attractive place.

When you first move your loved one out of your home, there is a deep sense of guilt, abandonment, and rejection that really never goes away. When I visited Phyllis, which was frequently (at least four to five times a week), I would have the same guilty feelings each time I skulked out of the assisted living facility.

My son Jared came down from New Jersey to help me move his mother in and was so upset at the thought of leaving her alone in this facility that he spent the first night in her suite on the couch. The move was an emotional one for all the family. There was also guilt and a constant feeling that I had abandoned my wife of over fifty years, but I was pleased that she was in such a pleasant place—and the staff assured me that they "would take care of her for life."

Tip: As mentioned, remote relatives always feel you have moved the loved one way too soon. However, most caregiving spouses and children move their loved ones too late as they are faced with the guilt and anguish of separation and other family resistance. If affordable, my advice is to move as soon as the loved one needs help with any of the life basics: dressing, bathing, grooming and hygiene, and transporting (walking) and is a danger of "eloping" (wandering). It's a very tough decision!

While some of the twenty-four patients had dementia problems, some only had various physical problems and were quite cogent. They also had a social or cocktail hour at five o'clock, which was a perfect visiting time for me and other visitors since we could gracefully leave after socializing, when they rolled the residents into six o'clock dinner. They offered real wine, nonalcoholic wine, and various juices. One ninety-seven-year-old lady would roll up each afternoon pushing her walker with a straight-up martini carefully balanced on the seat. One of the residents had a cute little dog named Rosie. Phyllis loved dogs and constantly followed and petted Rosie. One time, she accompanied Rosie and her owner on a walk around the grounds. Almost immediately, I received a call from the staff saying Phyllis was a candidate for "elopement."

"Good God!" I said. "With whom?"

The administrator said, to my relief, "No, you don't understand, elopement means the risk of roaming."

I asked what I should do about it.

"You either have to move her to a locked facility, especially for memory care, or if you want to keep her here, you will have to have a caregiver 24/7. We cannot risk the liability of having your wife wander off the property."

Well, here I thought I had found a place for Phyllis forever and almost completely covered by the $8,000 a month I received from long-term-care insurance, and now they were blithely telling me I would need to pay an estimated $20 an hour x 24/7, bringing my total non-reimbursed monthly outlay to $14,000 per month—over and above long-term-care coverage. This would mean that I have to lay out about $170,000 more a year than I had planned, which would cut drastically into my fixed monthly income from my investment portfolio, which we were largely living on. So much for "we will keep her for life."

ALF rough costs combined with full-time nursing

Basic ALF Cost	$ 8,000	per month
24/7 Nurse @ $20/hour	+ 14,400	per month
Total Cost	22,400	per month
Long-term Care Insurance	-8,000	per month
Net Cost	14,400	per month
My Out-of-Pocket	$170,400	per year

Note: Without insurance, the out-of-pocket would be $260,000 per year, which was prohibitive for me and most families.

Notes

Nursing Home II (Memory Care)

I quickly—probably too quickly—looked for the first memory care or "lock-up" unit. I put Phyllis into one for about three months until it was clear they were overmedicating the residents. At that point, I brought her home for eight months.

On a Sunday morning, I walked into Phyllis's (first) memory care facility (and second nursing home), and about thirty residents were sitting in a wide circle with their heads bowed.

How nice, I thought, a Sunday prayer service.

It didn't take me long to figure out they were not praying—they had been heavily Xanaxed and had zoned out.

The whole scene was so depressing that I brought Phyllis home and back to full-time home care for eight months, despite her declining condition and the need for even more care since increasing incontinence brought on urinary tract infections. Urinary tract infections are a common problem with Alzheimer's victims since they don't remember to go to the bathroom. If the staff doesn't check them frequently, they will be virtually sitting/lying in their own urine for hours.

In many ways, it was good to have her home. We managed with one excellent caregiver who could live in and not charge while she slept because she had the baby monitor.

My plan was to keep Phyllis home for eight months, at least through Christmas and New Year's while the kids were with us for the holidays. Right after the first of the year, I moved her to a third institution, a nearby memory care unit that was part of an assisted living facility. This, of course, involved another move, including furniture, rehanging pictures, transferring the virtually useless phone (she couldn't use or answer it), plus the community down payment and a month's fee in advance, more paperwork, qualifying the nursing home and its license, inspection of both Phyllis and the memory care unit by the long-term-care company, getting the administration to properly format and submit claims to the insurance company, and face another cash flow lag while waiting for insurance payments which, again, ran about four to five months in arrears if not correctly filed. Besides the financial aspects, the moves in and out of facilities and home made it a very pressure-laden year. Meanwhile, I had also moved from our larger house to a charming smaller house in a retirement community close to the first nursing home, creating further pressure on myself.

Tip: Check out assisted living facilities, especially "good-for-life" promises! Do not be surprised if the first facility is not your last one—as I assumed—unless they have a memory clinic for later-stage Alzheimer's disease. Even then, memory care was not our final stop.

Notes

Nursing Home III (Memory Care)

After Christmas and the holidays and visits from the kids, I moved Phyllis (January 2014) into the third facility, which was the second memory unit. This meant the patients/residents were locked in to prevent wandering. They did have access to a nice garden and enclosed walking paths, and Phyllis had a two-room suite (furnished by me, of course) and a bathroom for just under $5,000 a month.

This lock-up facility was a little lighter and brighter than the previous memory care facility, and the residents seemed to be more active and involved, as opposed to being totally zonked out or Xanaxed into oblivion as they had been in the previous place.

Phyllis was ambulatory and was able to talk to some of the more cogent residents. The new place was very close to my new house, and I would frequently take Phyllis out for lunch, especially to her favorite restaurant on the river where she could see a lot of boats and pelicans, and then I would bring her to my house where we would watch tennis or football together. I know she really couldn't follow a sitcom or drama, but she seemed okay with sports, nature films, game shows, and some of our grandchildren's favorite programs.

At some point, I realized taking Phyllis out to a restaurant and bringing her home to watch TV had a certain amount of denial for me as to her condition. There was also nostalgia as I tried to simulate aspects of the more normal half century we had lived together. When she visited, I had to stock the bathrooms at home with Depends. Phyllis would frequently wander around the new house aimlessly. She loved going outside—my patio abutted a golf course and a lake—to watch the birds. When planes flew overhead, she would frequently go out and wave her arms at the plane, absolutely certain that the pilot had seen her and that she was helping with his direction. She was quite confused about my new one-story house, which was loaded with familiar objects, paintings and pictures of her kids and family, which she welcomed but was very concerned about "the nonexistent lady upstairs." After each "date" together outside the walls of the home, I would have to strategically determine how to return her to the lock-up unit without her crying or begging me to come with her as they locked the door behind her.

Upon leaving, I would say something about having to drive somewhere to trick her into staying behind in the facility. Sometimes I told her I had some errands to run and would see her "in a bit." I have to advise, regrettably, that sometimes dissembling and redirecting are important parts of caregiving. I would often skulk away from the facility with feelings of guilt and tears welling up in my eyes. I certainly believe that I received more benefit from the meals out and watching television together at "home" than Phyllis, but I think, at some level, she got satisfaction from being with me and also appreciated our desperate need for short periods of "normalcy."

However, as Phyllis became more disoriented, the head nurse said our luncheon "dates" were probably too much for her. She suggested having future luncheons within the facility. She said, "Moving from the facility to the car, to the restaurant and back again, is far too much change for her—and disruptive." It also made my departure more difficult after her temporary sense of "freedom." Also, there was the disappointment as she assumed each visit I was there to "spring" her and take her "home" for good.

Notes

Nursing Home IV (Rehab)

To compound our problems of coping with Alzheimer's disease, I received an urgent call from the third home, the most recent memory care facility. They had sent Phyllis by ambulance to the ER. She had apparently taken a bad fall, and we later learned that her right hip was broken. It had to be partially replaced, and the home indicated they would not take her back unless she was ambulatory.

After Phyllis broke her hip and underwent a partial replacement, she was moved to the rehabilitation center, which was also considered an SNF (skilled nursing facility). This was her fourth place of residence in eighteen months. She occupied a large and quite expensive single room ($16,500/month), and they began physical therapy despite the fact that Phyllis would probably never be able to walk again. Financially, it was a big mistake because physical therapy was painful and was almost useless in her case. It was covered by Medicare—they paid the institution directly—while a long-term-care company informed me they would not recognize claims if they are being partially met by Medicare. Consequently, claims for the $675 per day were turned back by the long-term-care insurance company, while the payments for Phyllis's physical therapy were not deducted from my bill—despite the fact that the rehab had received the funds directly. As you might imagine, this presented a sizable cash-flow drain because the approximately $16,500 per month payments for Phyllis's room and care were not reimbursed one penny by our policy.

I eventually was able to move her to a cheaper single room for $12,500/month. Once I was able to suspend the physical therapy and get the administration office to correctly submit claims to the insurance company, payments started coming in. Since they were about five months late, I had to dip into another pot of cash resources to the tune of $70,000. Compounded with the prior year where the second nursing home had been unable to provide my long-term-care insurance company with sufficient paperwork for almost a year, I was down more than $140,000 in cash flow over those two calendar years. Meanwhile, the rehab, despite their claim for providing long-term-care patients, wanted to expel her for her pseudobulbar affect breakouts.

They knew at the rehab that we couldn't really leave the facility unless Phyllis had a place to go, and moving her was far more difficult than I thought. The rehab facility (desperate to get rid of her) and I, approached forty different memory care/nursing homes and were turned down by all of them with the exception of one that was 144 miles away. Apparently, once these facilities saw the medications she was taking, which included Xanax, Ativan, antipsychotics, and Nuedexta for pseudobulbar affect, and after each potential new "home" talked with the head nurse at the rehab facility, all of these places determined that Phyllis would be a major disturbance to their other patients.

In one of her last cogent sentences, Phyllis—in her wheelchair and with pain on her face—asked, "What did I do to deserve this?" Indeed!

Tip: Understand what Medicare covers and does not cover. Refer to Medicare.gov. No one warned me that Medicare, paying for the modest cost of physical therapy, might disqualify me from the $7,800/month coverage by my long-term-care policy.

My sister-in-law who lives in Cincinnati felt she had found a good facility there for memory care patients only, but I abhorred the idea of not being able to see Phyllis frequently, particularly while she still recognized me and felt I was some kind of link to reality for her and her former life.

Sarcastically, after an extensive search for a home to transfer Phyllis, I would comment that there must be some other people in the state of Florida who had symptoms similar to Phyllis's; therefore, there must be a suitable number of nursing homes. From the literature, I determined that Phyllis's behavior from her pseudobulbar affect was not that much outside the norm as Alzheimer's disease patients typically experience sundowners, hysterics, delusions, and spontaneous outbursts. Finding a place to transfer Phyllis was a time of desperation for me since there was a deadline for moving out of the rehab facility. The sadness the disease created for me and our extended family, the concern over finding the proper place for Phyllis, and the financial considerations all weighed heavily on me and exacerbated the dismal outlook we faced.

As in the case of the previous facilities, the application for my claims by the rehab were not processed on a timely basis, and my negative cash flow was a drag on my assets and increasing my debt. I quickly amassed more delayed claim payments. Hopefully, you will not have to change facilities as frequently as I did since each change required a nonreturnable placement fee and then a few months of lag until the long-term-care insurance claims were properly made and kicked on. I recognized I have made finances part of the story, but frankly, it is a sobering side effect of the disease.

At this juncture, you must realize that your work is likely not over once you have your loved one safely in a facility.

Just a word about skilled nursing facility and Medicare Part A services. To obtain this coverage, according to the Social Security Administration, your need must occur within thirty days of a hospital stay of at least three or more days. It must also be an extension of the treatment you receive for your hospitalized condition and require daily skilled nursing care as certified by your doctor. If you meet these conditions, Medicare will pay 100 percent of the first twenty days. For days twenty-one to one hundred, there is a hefty coinsurance payment per day for each benefit $164.50 (2017). After the hundred days, apparently all the costs are either on you or your long-term care if you have an LTC policy.

My Rehab Financial Costs

	Private Room	Insurance Pays (Long-Term Care) With Medicare	Without Medicare/ Physical Therapy
First Room	$16,500/ month	None	$7,800/ month
Second Room	$12,500/ month	None	$7,800/ month

Note: Medicare payments were for four hours of physical training per week and were paid directly to the rehab facility. Physical therapy costs were $400 per week, so my out-of-pocket during physical therapy was $12,000–$16,000 per month until I discontinued it. If Phyllis had qualified for a semiprivate room, these costs would have been greatly reduced.

With all of the institutions I moved Phyllis into, the initial claims were all sent back because they were not satisfactorily filled out. For example, one assisted living facility would submit February's bill at the end of February instead of March 1, and that one day was sufficient for the insurance company to return the claim indicating that payments of claims can only be made following completion of the month of service. So, if the institution had waited one day and submitted on March 1 instead of February 28, I would have been paid six to eight weeks sooner. Another had "change of personnel" and could not provide proper licensing approval for the long-term-care company until a year later. As I was spending quite a bit of time and capital on the paperwork involved in Phyllis's residences, I couldn't help wondering, when looking at all the other elderly residents:

1. Who would take care of them if they returned home?
2. Who would prepare the paperwork and follow up on the insurance claims?
3. In the event of a cash flow bind such as I faced, how would they handle bridging the gap? I maxed out a couple of credit cards to make my loose ends meet.

I am concerned that many spouses and family caregivers wouldn't have these financial options.

Regrettably, the impact of the disease, the discomfort of your loved one, the extensive paperwork, and the negative cash flow can be almost paralyzing.

A disclaimer: Please realize that our situation, compounded by the screaming effects of P.B.S. represented a very small percentage of AD patients and many families can usually find the appropriate facility and only need to place their loved one once. We were definitely a "worst case experience," and our personal tale is cautionary.

Notes

Nursing Home V
(Private Home Care)

I was just about at the end of my rope when my cousin suggested I talk to one of her friends whose brother-in-law had been in a caregiver's private home and was taken care of 24/7 by a caring, experienced individual who took only one patient at a time. My cousin's friend gave me a rave review about Sandy Streeter; her husband actually had been in Sandy's home for some period of time. The clincher was when she said, "When my time comes, I want to also be at Sandy's." I also heard of great references Sandy had from other people we knew, including the head of the local Alzheimer's center and one of Phyllis's college roommates.

Mine was hardly an unusual situation, and I wondered why this setup had not become a cottage industry for private in-home care long before. (Maybe it is, but it is not publicized very well.) As life expectancy grows, there must be a geometrical need for "warehousing" our elderly and infirmed.

The Sandy solution seemed like a perfect one, and Phyllis went to live in her home. She had her own spacious room and bath and was in calm surroundings. We were relieved at this solution.

Sandy's daughter was a licensed professional nurse, which meant she could dispense the meds. Phyllis's favorite feature was Sandy's fourteen-month-old African American grandchild who Phyllis figured was one of her own grandchildren. Sandy lived close enough to me that I was able to easily visit Phyllis four or five times per week. When Phyllis wasn't in bed, she was in a comfortable recliner in Sandy's living room. She could watch TV and be involved in the comings and goings of three generations of Sandy's family; it was a good arrangement until Sandy's daughter took Phyllis's daily blood pressure—and it recorded 45 over 0. They immediately called 911 to get her to the hospital.

Notes

Death–Hospice

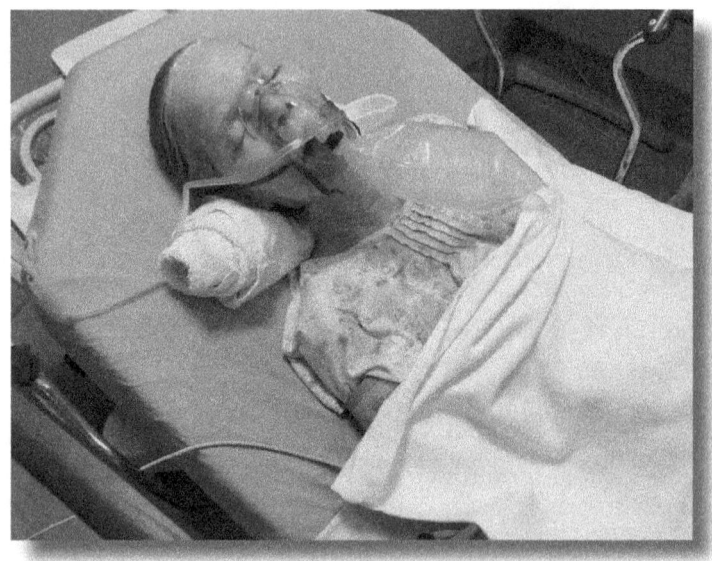

Phyllis

In the very late stages of Alzheimer's disease, the victim could have a number of causes for their final death. Unfortunately, these include a number of not-so-desirable symptoms that result directly or indirectly from Alzheimer's, such as a complete decline in the immune system, which can lead to pneumonia or other inflammatory diseases. Frequently,

Alzheimer's disease victims begin to have trouble swallowing and lose other motor reflexes, which can cause them considerable discomfort and pain.

Medical doctors have traditionally been instilled with the tenants of the Hippocratic oath, which states, "Do no harm," but the physician may take whatever steps are necessary to extend the lives of their patients, irrespective of the quality of that extended life, unless restrained by legal concerns. Fortunately, when my moment of truth came in the ER, I had read *Being Mortal* by Dr. Atul Gawande. He is a strong advocate of palliative care at the end of life. He states, "Nasogastric tubes are uncomfortable, tortuous devices." These tubes are placed through the nose and into the gastrointestinal tract to the stomach for feeding and medication.

The purpose of palliative care is to provide maximum comfort during the end days. It is thankfully a growing segment of medicine since I cannot imagine anything worse than extending a life that has no quality and is frequently uncomfortable if not "torturous."

The palliative approach consists of painkillers, other comfort-promoting medications, and even a morphine drip when needed.

When I received a call from Sandy, Phyllis's blood pressure had been relatively normal the night before, but it had apparently plunged by morning. By the time I got to the ER, Phyllis was already there with a large oxygen mask over her face. Several physicians were trying to revive her. The ER physician asked me over the noise of the machines and the medical assistants if I wanted to intubate her, which could provide nourishment and possibly extend her life a few hours or even a day or two. I said no and indicated I wanted her sent to a hospice house ASAP. The doctor said that he doubted that she would last long enough to get there.

When we first arrived at the hospice house, they furnished me with a booklet called *Gone from My Sight* by Barbara Karnes, which gave me a pretty good orchestration of the dying experience. Although I thought the dying experience varied greatly with individuals, it was apparently not always the case, especially in a hospice house. Some parts that applied to Phyllis's situation were as follows:

- A couple of months before her death, we saw a definite withdrawal from the world, and her food intake decreased.
- A couple of weeks before, there was further disorientation and confusion accompanied by decreased blood pressure and becoming pale. She was sleeping most of the time, but she

could respond momentarily if awakened or greeted. Her blood pressure, which had been low for several months, was going even lower. Her interest in eating was waning.

- A week before her death, she was totally disoriented and not communicating.
- Just a couple of days before her death, her eyes became glassy and half-open. The nurse told her she could probably not see us, but she could hear what we were saying as we talked openly in front of her. Her skin was further paling, and there was mottling in some areas, such as the extremities. Her blood pressure was further declining, and her breathing became irregular, even stopping for several seconds at times.
- Hours and minutes before her death, her breathing slowed, and there was an occasional pause, then gasping, but she didn't appear at all uncomfortable.

We couldn't arouse or awaken her to talk to her, and her breathing declined. Finally, except for a couple of deep breaths, it stopped entirely.

It appeared to me that her last days were comfortable, calm, and painless. It also seemed there was a clear transition from the physical world she had lived in all her life to existence on a more spiritual plane. I climbed into bed with her and held her during the last minutes of her life. I told her how much I loved her, who was there, and how much each of them loved her. I thought I could actually feel the spirit leaving her now-lifeless body.

In sum, I was very glad that I had scoped out the hospice house well in advance. The staff was very attentive and helpful, the setting was tranquil, and the transition from life to death went as smoothly and comfortably as possible.

Tip: There is also hospice care available in your home, in the hospital, or even in the care receiver's nursing home. The closer your loved one is to death, the more hospice can help—and the less it costs. In extremis, Medicare pays for it all, in my experience.

Grim as death is, the hospice house was a great help for both Phyllis's physical comfort and the family's emotional comfort.

Phyllis

How Do I Love Thee?
(Sonnet 43)

How do I love thee? Let me count the ways.
I love thee with the breath,
smiles, tears, of all my life;
And, if God choose,
I shall but love thee better after death.

—Elizabeth Barrett Browning (1806–1861)

Ode on Intimations of Immortality

Thanks to the human heart by which we live,
Thanks to its tenderness, its joys, and fears,
To me the meanest flower that blows can give
Thoughts that do often lie too deep for tears.

—William Wordsworth (1770–1850)

Notes

Loss

The loss of a loved one can certainly be one of the most traumatic events in a person's life. When the services are over, the burial has taken place, and the funeral flowers have wilted, a huge hole remains in your heart. Most of us soldier on and live our lives, but we are always conscious on some level of our own personal tragedy and the acute loss of a dear one. Sudden loss can be a shock to your entire system, to your way of life, to your faith, and to your thinking for the rest of your life. Slow loss can be almost worse since the Alzheimer's disease patient dies a little every day. I lost my mother when I was eighteen, and I still miss her terribly, decades later. I see her constantly somewhere in the so-called mind's eye.

Irrespective of your beliefs or lack of same, the passing of a loved one continues to impact and shape your thought processes. Then there is death by a thousand cuts. That is Alzheimer's. Over the past ten years, I had seen a little bit of Phyllis slip away until she became a nonperson. There are no surprises here; the books warned me that such a decline would take place. However, in the stark reality of day-to-day life, you are always in a state of day-to-day mourning. Initially, you notice the symptoms you have read about: the loss of the keys, the seeking a substitute word when she can't recall the appropriate one, growing difficulties with the simplest tasks, and forgetting.

You still have conversations increasingly about the children or other family members and less about world events as her "universe" implodes. Just two years ago, at the dinner table with new friends or new acquaintances, I observed Phyllis exuberantly talking to the people on her right and left. You watch their faces as they are engaged by this lovely, outgoing woman. Then you will see gradual consternation forming on their faces as they start trying to unravel some of Phyllis's non sequiturs. At that point, they begin to nod a lot. Initially, her comments may sound rational, but as it sinks in, you'll miss a key word or two that makes the whole comment questionable if not incomprehensible. The kinder seatmates attempt to continue some thread of what they are talking about, but even they give up when they realize she is talking in phrases without syntax. During the mild stage of Phyllis's disease, I would usually ask the host to inform the guests that Phyllis was in the early stage of Alzheimer's and to bear with her.

In the middle stages of her disease, I frankly had to regret party and dinner invitations, and Phyllis's circle of friends was limited to a very few good ones she'd known for decades. In the late, mid-advanced stage, there were no dinners and cocktail parties, and our social activity was limited to the few good friends and having a sandwich or a drink with them, plus holidays with our kids and grandkids.

Although I knew we were on an inevitable downward slide health-wise, every now and then Phyllis, would have a good day that would falsely prop up my hopes. But the inevitable was the inevitable, and the uneven downward descent would be much like following the downticks of the Dow Jones average in a recession. While still at home, there would be little mini tragedies such as the day she could no longer put on her pajamas or the day that she could no longer brush her teeth. I was relieved of a lot of these responsibilities when we moved Phyllis to assisted living, but that presented another great emotional barrier for me to leap. As I repeatedly mentioned, the sense of abandonment and guilt as you leave your loved one behind a locked door each visit further compounds the growing sense of loss.

Every now and then, I think that I would pay almost anything to go back in time and have only one more day (or even one hour) with a cogent Phyllis—to be able to talk to her, converse with her, hug her, and have her recognize me. I am not sure how much I would tell her about her future bout with Alzheimer's, but if we could reminisce and be husband and wife on normal terms for just half an hour, it would be a marvelous gift anytime, but especially in the end days. During that half hour, her sense of humor would return, her physical loveliness would be restored, her love of her children would be as poignant as it's ever been, and I would hold and kiss her "not as a stranger." Sometimes it is difficult to remember just how the person was when they were normal because they become so inarticulate and helpless that they start to take on the foggy identity of another person or, more accurately, a nonperson.

At Phyllis's funeral, my daughter CeCe read a touching poem about having "one more day" with her mother. How often I wish I could talk to Phyllis for a day or even an hour when she was functioning normally. I frequently would like to ask her a question or bounce an idea or discuss the kids and their progress—or even just get a hug.

I really could not say or measure how the death of the "long goodbye" compares with a sudden death or how the expected is any easier than the unexpected. Both are tragic inflection points in our lives.

In these days of paying practically only lip service to a higher authority, I feel that my ordeal with Phyllis's Alzheimer's disease brought me closer to God, and it gave me a greater knowledge of my own strengths and weaknesses.

Before Alzheimer's disease, my life had not been characterized by patience, helping others, care, or prayer. I had not spent much time considering disease or death; they were distant abstracts and so were the concepts of heaven and hell. I would go through the motions of attending church with the family, but my prayers were mundane and too often usually self-serving.

Looking back over Phyllis's long decline, I have to say my life objectives took a sharp turn, as did my ranking of those elements of life that are most important. This evolution was not a sudden light on the road to Damascus. Initially, I questioned how such a good person as Phyllis could be subjected to such a cruel fate. Then I petitioned God to make her as comfortable as possible on this earth and then to take her to her rightful place in heaven. I held no bizarre hopes that Phyllis would ever recover, but I did want her time on this earth to be free of fear, pain, and worry.

During this long process, as you may have gathered, I also started feeling a little sorry for myself: having household responsibilities thrust upon me that had been carried by Phyllis, carrying the burden of Phyllis's several moves from one facility to another, ambulances racing her to the ER initially with a sprained neck and secondly a broken hip, coordinating doctors, moving furniture several times in one year, and interfacing with insurance companies. I was slowly losing my wife, and the unforeseen process of losing her was overwhelming me on physical, emotional, and financial levels. What saved me from counseling aid was a few Xanax and the growing belief in God's endgame for a person as good, generous, and loving as Phyllis. As I said at our fiftieth wedding anniversary party, without any exaggeration, "She was lovely both outside and in." I got to say that again at her funeral.

Notes

My Funeral Comments

July 27, 2016

This has been a long and heavy cross to bear for me and my children, grandchildren, Phyllis's siblings, and all who knew and loved her. Our family's loss is unquantifiable. We all watched this dear person fade and die a little every day from the scourge of Alzheimer's—a terrible disease for both victim and caregiver.

In the many cards and communications I received, almost everyone talks about Phyllis's beauty, kindness, warmth, openness, and love of her family. She had an immutable faith in God and never, never questioned the existence of heaven—where she will undoubtedly be an "early-admissions candidate."

She was lovely both outside and in, never judgmental or prejudiced. She was kind to all and raised our children with the same principles she lived by:

- love for one another
- forgive every trespass

- love our country
- love our family
- above all, love the Lord our God

The only consolation that we have is that she passed in relative comfort surrounded by her family before the onset of cruel late-stage symptoms. I can only thank God for bringing this beautiful being into my life. She steadied me, gave me faith, gave me children, and gave me her unconditional love—all better than I deserved.

Goodbye for now, sweetie. I know I will be with you again when my time comes. We will all remember you and love you *always*. I miss you dreadfully! As the poet said, "Death be not proud!"

Raleigh Coffin

A Parable of Immortality

I am standing upon the seashore.
A ship at my side spreads her white
sails to the morning breeze
and starts for the blue ocean.

She is an object of beauty and strength,
and I stand and watch until at last she hangs
like a speck of white cloud
just where the sea and sky come
down to mingle with each other.
Then someone at my side says,
"There, she is gone!"
"Gone where?"

Gone from my sight. That is all.
She is just as large in mast and hull and spar
as she was when she left my side
and just as able to bear her load of living freight
to her destined port.

Phyllis

Her diminished size is in me, not in her.
And just at the moment
when someone at my side says:
"There, she is gone!"
There are other eyes watching her coming,
and other voices ready to take up the glad shout:
"Here she comes!"
And that is dying.

—Henry Van Dyke

Notes

Appendix A: Medical Advances

Frankly, the prospect for the near-term availability of a cure for Alzheimer's looks pretty dim for all but one or two promising approaches as described below. As of this writing (2018), there has been very little progress on the medical front. In fact, Eli Lilly has just spent more than $1 billion on their experimental drug Solanezumab, which is designed for attacking clumps of protein that are called beta-amyloids. The company indicated that it would not seek regulatory approval to market this experimental medication because it didn't significantly slow down or "cure" cognitive decline in patients. This is just one of the several attempts by pharmaceutical companies to attack beta-amyloid hypothesis without any resounding success.

Another school of experimentation is designed to attack tau proteins, which can form tangles that are destructive to brain cells. As I write, companies including J&J, Roche, Bristol-Myers, and AbbVie, Inc. are developing drugs that target tau. However, one of the most promising tau drugs (LMTM) has recently failed to show much of an effect. The competitive camps for attacking beta-amyloid versus tau proteins seem to be somewhat divided.

Rakez Kayed, a neuroscientist, said, "Going after plaques alone probably isn't the best strategy and would seem that combination therapy targeting several Alzheimer's-related proteins could be more productive."

I personally hope that these camps can come together and try a full-court assault on the disease rather than driving down a single-lane road.

Another obvious conclusion is that they could be possibly more successful if they treated the disease much earlier—before the start of the symptoms. To me, this creates a conundrum because how do you know you have the disease unless there are some symptoms?

It would seem, when reading the literature, that we are at a very primitive stage in dealing with diseases of the brain, and much of the challenge could be a function of the scientists' incomplete understanding of the role of the beta-amyloid, tau, and possibly other destructive proteins and their interactions.

Meanwhile, pharmaceutical firms are pursuing hundreds of different treatments, and even the most advanced won't be showing test results until 2018 to

2020 or beyond. On the promising side, it appears that we will be able to make earlier determinations of the presence of the disease through DNA diagnosis, providing evidence of a proclivity toward developing the disease. Challenging the progress on the early diagnosis is the fact that many cognitively "healthy" people also have amyloids present in their brains, and one of the key factors will be to identify what factors trigger or create the destructive amyloids, thereby creating Alzheimer's and other dementia diseases such as Lewy body disease.

The report card on experimental success for Alzheimer's disease has been close to failing. In fact, the experimental failure rate, according to the *Wall Street Journal,* is 99.6 percent since 2004, while the failure rate of oncology research is 81 percent. Additionally, in the United States, we spend $215 billion per year on Alzheimer's disease versus $100 billion on heart-related diseases and $77 billion for cancer. Currently, Alzheimer's constitutes 20 percent of the total Medicare/Medicaid budget and is spent on research, most of which has been targeted on the beta-amyloid hypothesis. Unless there is some medical breakthrough in the next couple of decades, Alzheimer's disease could top $1 trillion by 2050 for treatment and care.

Hopefully, recently passed legislation (the 21st Century Cures Act) will accelerate pinpoint diagnosis based on the individual's genome and speed up the laborious approval process.

Genetic Research

An important part of Alzheimer's research is determining how the Alzheimer's beta-amyloids are passed on genetically. That factor, of course, is of great concern to my family as it would appear they could have a 50 percent chance of developing Alzheimer's in later years unless preventive pharmaceuticals are discovered or created in the near future.

While giant strides have been made in the field of genetic diagnosis and therapy for all disease victims, the projections for AD inheritance is still pretty general. Conventional wisdom says that if one parent contracted AD, your chance of becoming an AD victim is 50 percent.

The more family members who are affected by AD, the greater your risk. Apparently, an estimated 25 percent of AD patients have a definite family history of the disease. These are sketchy generalities because the medical industry has yet to find the specific gene mutation responsible for AD. However, there is least one suspicious culprit or gene variant at this writing that would appear to increase the propensity for contracting the disease: ApoE4.

Researchers do not think that ApoE4 directly causes AD, but it increases the loss of nerve cell functioning and "ages" the brain at a faster rate.

Why not test everybody for this gene variant? Although large-scale testing has associated ApoE4 with a slowed brain development, not all AD victims have the ApoE4 gene—and not all those who carry the gene have or will have AD. Therefore, testing for ApoE4 alone is not practical at this time. Also, this gene variant is not the sole gene that contributes to cognitive decline, but its presence can infer a higher risk for carriers than those without the ApoE4 present.

Although genetic research is very promising, it is in very early stages and is only one of the many directions that need to be explored.

Other Research Prospects

The main reason that Alzheimer's disease requires so much more expenditure is that the victims sooner or later will require total care either in the home or in some manner of nursing home, possibly for years.

Alzheimer's disease is a neurodegenerative disorder that robs memory, independent living, and eventually the lives of 5.4 million Americans—and growing—each year. One estimate indicated there will be as many as 25 million victims by 2050. Assuming each victim affects the lives, time, and finance of at least five family members and friends, it would mean at least one-third of the total American population would be involved in the care and support of loved ones. This is a pandemic-like consequence.

At least one hopeful pharmaceutical prospect being tested will slow the disease's progress, and in some cases, it has actually reversed Alzheimer's by clearing the amyloid plaques from the brain. This product has been created and is being tested by Biogen. An interesting background story made the innovation possible. Several years ago, Dr. Chet Mathis of the University of Pittsburgh—in collaboration with Vienna's Dr. William Klunk and several other scientists—designed a "contrast agent" that could be safely injected and would travel to the brain of living (in vivo) Alzheimer's disease victims in X-rays, MRIs, and PET scans (positron emission tomography) to reveal the presence and location of the brain's plaques. Previously, such identification could only be achieved by postmortem autopsy.

This breakthrough could conceivably identify the disease at its early stages so that medical research might be able to encounter Alzheimer's disease earlier and slow or stop its progress.

The invention of Vizamyl was first presented to the medical profession in 2003. However, at that time, neither the FDA nor Medicare saw any value in the "contrast agent" because it did not treat the underlying cause of the disease. It was not until 2012 that the FDA finally gave approval, and today, the ability to track beta-amyloid plaques far earlier has led to the development of BIIB-037 and possibly many other "cures" for this pernicious tragic disease.

BIIB-037 is an active antibody, which once introduced to the brain—and with help from the brain's existing white blood cells—seizes and dissolves the plaque clumps and allegedly could return the patient to normal cognitive ability within a year. In early, limited human trials, it proved safe for 98 percent of the patients tested, and it has already proven effective in reducing amyloids in animal brains. In 2016, the FDA gave this drug "fast-track status." The drug is being subjected to more extensive trials that are currently in progress.

Obviously the unforeseen can take place, which is the case with many new drug trials (see Eli Lily above). However, if the drug proves safe and effective, there will soon be the considerable hope for victims in the early stages of Alzheimer's disease and those who contract the disease in the future.

Other Research Areas
<u>AD Vaccines</u>

AD vaccines are also being aggressively evaluated, and they could possibly clear plaques from the brain by using the patient's own immune system or injecting antibodies to create an immune response in the patient.

<u>Fluselenamyl</u>

There is also a not yet approval for a compound called Fluselenamyl, which potentially can detect diffuse amyloid plaques, make imaging tests more valuable for early diagnosis of Alzheimer's disease, and monitor response to AD treatment.

The above are just a few of the cures and testing being currently pursued. Obviously, any "cures" will be too late for my wife and advanced stage AD victims, but for my kids and millions of others, there is at least a glimmer of hope that this pernicious disease will be conquered in the next few years.

Notes

Appendix B: Diet

Remember to Eat—but Eat to Remember

In addition to the fairly standard prescription drugs provided by neurologists mentioned above (Aricept, Exelon Patch, Namenda, etc.), there appear to be major breakthroughs in diet alone that can reduce the risk of developing or slowing Alzheimer's to a large extent. In 2015, new clinical studies have shown some alleged reversals of cognitive dysfunction, particularly in the elderly, of up to 50 percent when they follow recommended dietary habits. A new diet called MIND was developed from a long-established Mediterranean and DASH (Dietary Approaches to Stop Hypertension) diets. To oversimplify, the MIND diet emphasizes the following brain healthy food groups:

- green leafy vegetables
- other vegetables
- nuts

- berries (especially strawberries and blueberries)
- beans
- whole grains
- fish
- poultry
- olive oil
- wine (especially red ones)
- green tea

The study conducted by Hunt University also outlined the five "dangerous" food groups that are generally huge parts of the American diet and constitute some of our favorite meals. As strict compliance with the MIND diet (Mediterranean-DASH intervention for Neurodegenerative Delay) requires considerable discipline, there is some leeway provided for limited inclusion of "bad" foods such as:

- red meats—less than four servings per week
- butter/oleo margarine—less than one tablespoon per week
- cheese—less than one serving per week
- pastries/sweets—less than five servings per week
- fried fast foods—less than one serving per week

Although the above may seem unreasonably strict for our type of living, they nevertheless have had astonishing results in reducing the incidence of contracting Alzheimer's disease in the first place and have also shown favorable results for early- to mid-stage victims. In fact, in the Hunt study, people who carefully and dutifully pursued MIND showed a significant 52 percent reduction in the rate of developing Alzheimer's disease versus those who complied the least. As a side benefit, the diet should also help control blood pressure, weight, carbs, and reduce risk of heart attack and stroke.

In addition to the above, certain dietary supplements including CoQ10, melatonin, polyphenols, magnesium, vitamin D3, and resveratrol provide for further protection from contracting Alzheimer's disease and reduction in the decline of cognitive ability. I am sure in the years ahead, diet and supplements will be further defined and new nutritional combinations will be discovered, but so far, the nutritional balance provided by both diet and supplements seems to outstrip the prospects of cures provided by pharmaceutical companies and basic Alzheimer's research, and they should be given considerable emphasis among Alzheimer's disease patients, their children, and healthy people who want to protect their minds.

Turmeric (Curcumin)

I am not qualified nor is the purpose of this book to provide nutritional advice. However, I do think there are a few key foods/nutrients that can be easily assimilated into your daily diet that could provide you with a tremendous defense against contracting Alzheimer's—and maybe even slowing if not reversing the disease among those already affected.

The first of these is curcumin. Statistics of India indicate that there are only 4.4 million cases of Alzheimer's disease in this country versus 5.4 million in our country, despite the fact that we have a quarter of their population.

As you probably know, there is huge consumption of curry in India. In fact, Indian foods are characterized by various types of curry, which contain the spice turmeric (curcumin). I'm not recommending that you have to eat out at an Indian restaurant several times a week. Turmeric (curcumin) is readily available in concentrated form as an over-the-counter product and is available in most pharmacies.

Amazingly the medical industry and the National Cancer Institute, after years of study, are starting to appreciate the powers of curcumin and its ready availability, combined with low cost, low toxicity, and high effectiveness in benefiting cancer patients.

It has been coined as the "ideal chemopreventative agent." It would be somewhat ironic if we found out that two of the great scourges of this country could be reversed and largely cured by this simple spice.

Despite the modern world's focus over the last century on patented chemical compound solutions, we should also be looking in God's vast laboratory for natural cures.

Green Tea (Mata)

However, if you wanted to skip all the above (not recommended) and just ingest arguably the most effective defense against the formation of amyloids, consider the enormous benefits of green tea consumption.

Some medical research has recently focused on the benefits of green tea for Alzheimer's disease and have isolated EGCG* as a possible beneficial factor present in green tea. Today, there are almost six thousand published tests on the broad health benefits of green tea. Many of these have long been known, but recent attention has focused on its potential to prevent and possibly reverse the onslaught

* EGCG (epigallocatechin) a beneficial polyphenol component, plus a powerful antioxidant.harmful plaques. In their place, it creates brand-new neurons in the brain (neurogenesis).

of Alzheimer's and other forms of dementia. They are finding that green tea actually attacks existing amyloids and prevents the formation of new

Green tea has been tested and shown to reduce the chances of contracting Alzheimer's disease by 54 percent in animals. To maximize the benefits, you would have to drink or consume the equivalent of seven to ten cups of green tea a day—each cup containing about 50 milligrams of green tea.

Fortunately, there are over-the-counter concentrated capsules, each containing the equivalent of 500–750 milligrams or ten to fifteen cups of green tea. These are provided by a number of well-known vitamin/nutrient suppliers and can be purchased online or by phone. Big Pharma has yet to come up with any known prescription drug that effectively prevents or reverses Alzheimer's disease. Green tea may provide a lot of the answers, but since it is not patentable, it may be given short shrift by pharmaceutical companies.

Green tea has shown to be effective with:

- repair of DNA
- restoring cells to help in reducing inflammation (and is present in so many diseases, particularly those affecting seniors)
- prostate cancer

- cardiovascular diseases
- squamous cell carcinomas
- breast cancer
- lung cancer
- obesity/body weight
- lipid clearance
- glucose
- cell division

Olive Oil

Extra virgin olive oil has been one of the mainstays of the Mediterranean diet, which has been proved useful in weight-loss regimens. Its positive effects have been largely due to its high content of monounsaturated fatty acids and polyphenols. It is a strong antioxidant and is fights inflammation.

Tip: More than three-quarters of commercial olive oils on the grocery shelves are adulterated or counterfeit. The words extra virgin, unfiltered, and cold-pressed should be clearly visible on the label.

In addition to olive oil's salutary effect on the cardiovascular system, it also reduces inflammation, which is blamed by many for almost all human diseases, and may inhibit Alzheimer's.

All three of the above (resveratrol, curcumin, and green tea) are available over the counter in concentrated capsule form.

For maximum protection against the onslaught of Alzheimer's and many other diseases, the MIND diet reinforced with the above OTC products should be employed by everyone seeking good health maintenance and cognitive retention.

Recently introduced to the market is algae oil, which apparently is higher in monounsaturated fats than olive oil, and it has a neutral flavor. I haven't tried it yet and can't recommend it, but it sounds healthy and better tasting.

Note: Any nutritional diet or medication mentioned herein should be cleared by your medical professional before using.

Notes

Notes

Appendix C: Medical Directives

One of the critical meetings at the men's association at the Alzheimer's disease center was the subject of *medical directives*. We were urged by a specialist to immediately obtain a power of attorney (POA) for the Alzheimer's disease patient. This is critical for being able to control your loved one's needs, final arrangements, expenses, and ultimate plan for "end of life." Your doctor should also have an existing DNR (do not resuscitate), and if your spouse or loved one is institutionalized, I advise having a DNH (do not hospitalize without permission from POA) so that a nursing home cannot ship her off to a hospital without your approval for perhaps some very unsavory life-extending procedures.

When Phyllis fell and broke her hip in 2015, I obviously approved them sending her to the emergency room and ultimately having hip replacement. There is a difference between providing comfort procedures for a patient and uncomfortable and oftentimes useless life-extending procedures. I urge you to see a lawyer, particularly an "eldercare" lawyer, to obtain:

- A durable POA is generally a close family member.
- Your living will, which covers the documentation you should have for final days and whatever state health directives you need so you can make the call when your loved one no longer has the quality of life to prevent a prolonged, painful, or uncomfortable existence.
- A health care surrogate—if not mentioned in the living will. While these are usually the POA, there may be a need for a more knowledgeable friend, family member, or even medical professional to make objective health decisions, especially if the family members are conflicted about "life-ending" alternatives.

Alzheimer's Disease Advanced Directives

Tip: As soon as possible, prepare your advanced directives.

Advanced directives will protect you, your loved one, and your family. The main components of these directives include:

A Living Will or Declaration

Although some states permit holographic (handwritten) wills, your best course of action is to employ an attorney and have your documents prepared by a professional who is aware of both federal and your home state laws. Parties must be capable and competent to sign.

The primary advantage of a living will is that it will provide you with protection and assurance that you or your loved one's wishes during end of life will be followed. For example, if you become incapable of providing informed consent for medical decisions, your wishes as to life-prolonging procedures will be carried out. If your doctor—in some states, two doctors are required—determines that you are in a persistent vegetative state or a terminal or end-stage condition, he or she can call a cessation of those life-prolonging procedures, which could be very uncomfortable and even painful for the patient, extending a very poor quality of life for sometimes as little as hours and, at the most, weeks.

This would not preclude the administration of medicine or procedures required to provide comfort or care or to alleviate pain. In your living will, it is advisable to name a "health care surrogate," usually the spouse or a competent member of the family to consult with the doctor for what can be very difficult and emotional decisions.

When I was summoned to the ER due to Phyllis's plunge in blood pressure, the ER doctor told me she was dying and asked if I wanted to intubate her, which would allow them to provide her with some nutrients. As I mentioned in my discussion of palliative medicine, intubation can be a "torturous" procedure.

I declined and requested that they immediately move Phyllis to a hospice house in order to provide her with maximum comfort in the remaining hours of her life. She received care and pain relief through medication and morphine drips.

Tip: Obviously, the living will should be prepared as soon as possible while both the care receiver and the health care surrogate are in a competent state of mind. Your family cannot prepare a living will for you once you are incompetent. In this case, your lawyer will recommend a health care proxy, which can be anyone competent, usually in this preferable order of selection:

- *spouse*
- *parent*
- *adult sibling*

- *adult relative*
- *close friend*
- *guardian ad litem (by the court)*

Durable Power of Attorney

This essential document outlines the powers the designee can perform on your behalf, including:

- consent to medical, therapeutic, and surgical procedures
- approval of drug administration
- financial matters: paying bills, selling/buying property, including real estate, stocks, and bonds, and submitting insurance claims.

Again, the POA should be prepared by a competent and preferably a personal attorney who knows something about you, your lifestyle, and your relationships.

Note: The healthcare surrogate and the power of attorney can be the same person, but if they are different individuals, the POA should be more familiar with family affairs since his or her involvement will probably be much greater than the surrogate's involvement. For example, when Phyllis was mentally sound, we had living wills prepared naming each other as both surrogate and POA. This was fortunate in that I had to use her POA multiple times, including some of the following:

- selling our jointly owned house when I downsized
- paying her bills and monitoring her accounts
- approving her hip replacement surgery
- closing her bank and credit card accounts
- providing directives such as DNR (do not resuscitate) and DNH (do not hospitalize without my consent)
- hospice care
- implementing her last wishes, including end-of-life decisions
- last rites, burial/cremation decisions (before her death)

Note: Since the POA and surrogate expire upon death, postmortem wishes should be clarified in advance, including religious preferences, burial location, special gifts (if not stipulated in the will), and any other last wishes. For more information, see comments on hospice and palliative medicine. Authorization to release protected health information should be signed so doctors and institution can have access to the patient's medical records, as required by HIPAA (The Health Insurance Portability and Accountability Act).

I had only casual discussions with Phyllis over the years about death and handling of remains. At a family meeting (my kids and her sisters) just days before her death, the point was made that as a young girl, she was taught in her catechism that a body should remain whole and not be cremated. The theory behind this was that our bodies joined our souls in heaven. (Why I or anybody would want an aged, decrepit body to join your essence for eternity escapes me.) Therefore, the "family" decided that she should be buried whole—except for her brain, which was shipped to the Mayo Clinic for analysis. It indicated she died primarily from Alzheimer's disease, but there was also a presence of Lewy body disease. Most religions (including Catholicism) now believe cremation is perfectly acceptable as our carnal bodies will not play a role in eternity—"dust to dust." Many believe our spirits will rise to be joined with new, eternal physical or metaphysical "presences" that transcend any form we know or could imagine.

Notes

References

Act Against Alzheimer's Disease. (n.d.). Retrieved from actionalz.org

Advanced Directives, Prestige Printing, Oviedo, F.

Alzheimer's Disease. (2012–17). Mount Sinai School of Medicine.

Cremens, M. Cornelia., MD, MPH (Ed.). (2017). *Combating Memory Loss*. Massachusetts General Hospital.

Final Wishes Planning Guide, Americo, Dallas, TX.

Gawande, A. (2014). *Being Mortal: Medicine and What Matters in the End*. New York: Metropolitan Books, Henry Holt and Company.

Genova, L. (2009). *Still Alice*. New York: Pocket Books.

Karnes, B. (2014). *Gone from My Sight: The Dying Experience*. Vancouver, WA: Barbara Karnes Books.

Mace, N. L., & Rabins, P. V. (2011). *The 36-Hour Day: A Family Guide to Caring for People Who Have Alzheimer Disease, Related Dementias, and Memory Loss.* Baltimore: Johns Hopkins University Press.

Also, many magazine articles, newsletters, pamphlets, and medical conferences.

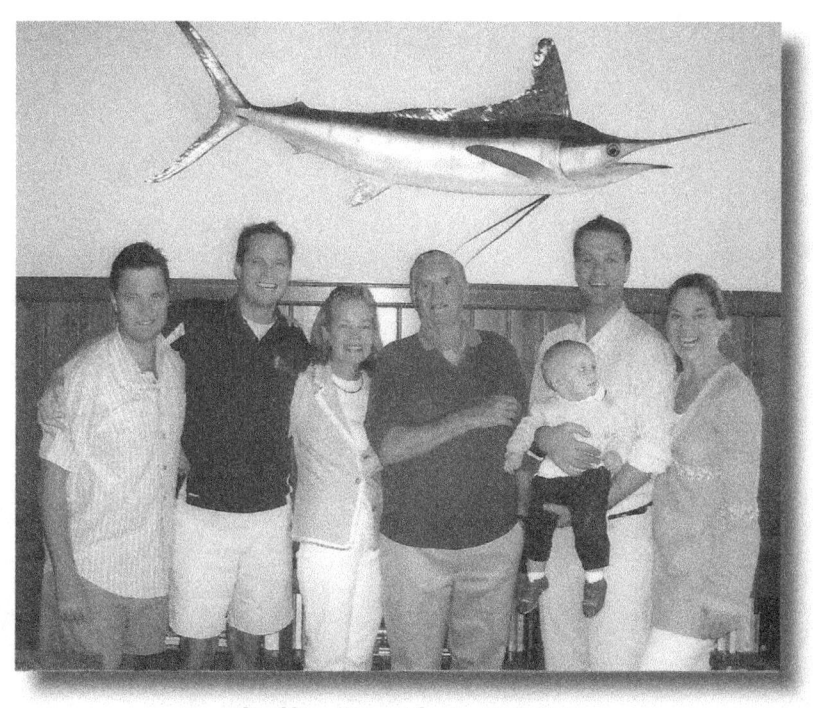

Coffin Family in 2007

Afterword

In reading over this work, I find it is almost a guide for what not to do. I would hope you would learn from my lessons, including:

1. Don't put an Alzheimer's disease patient into an assisted living facility unless they have a memory care unit.
2. Don't believe the nursing homes when they say, "We can keep your loved one for life." I found, in most cases, this not to be true—even in nursing homes with skilled nursing facilities.
3. Check further if they say they are temporarily shorthanded—since when and until when? In most homes, this was the case. The supply of nursing home workers is not keeping up with the demand of the nursing homes.
4. If you and your spouse are healthy and farsighted enough, check out continuing care retirement communities for lifelong continuing care. This would be the best and least

expensive alternative. Of course, most people cannot foresee the onslaught of the golden years early enough to make these kinds of plans.

5. Also, long-term care, which I foresee will be increasingly expensive over the years, needs foresight and planning. Remember, most of us will experience some form of disease, mental, problems or functional problems that will require at least short-term care—if not long-term care—in a facility. As medicine increases life expectancy, a greater percentage of seniors will require some form of institutional warehousing.

6. I've also spent a good deal of time on finances, which in my case, added considerably to the emotional pressure from my wife's condition. I apologize for this since it may add additional worries to your forthcoming situation, but it can be quite important if not done right. I think I am a classic example of someone who didn't do it right. Again, I hope my particular financial situation will be far worse than the one you will confront.

7. If you are a caregiver, I wish you the best and hope you undertake this experience with as little pressure as possible, such as

using outside help (including family if they are close by), and that you will be generous with your respites and breaks. Initially I felt guilty about taking time off away from my wife, but I would later come to realize that a day, a week, or even a month away recharged my batteries and helped me get through the days or weeks of repetitious routine.

8. In sum, Alzheimer's disease is not a good way to cap off you or your care receiver's life. Tragically, things do not get better. As a caregiver is constantly under pressure, duress, and emotional sadness, you may want to seek out professional help to provide feedback and supportive medicine.

God bless all caregivers. They are drafted into one of the most selfless and sacrificial periods of their lives. May their care receivers experience minimal discomfort and depression and experience the most loving care possible.

As one health provider on a CBS documentary reported, "I married for better or for worse, but Alzheimer's disease is worse than worse."

—Raleigh Coffin
Vero Beach, Florida
April 2018

In Appreciation

Despite the fact that I have made myself out to be some kind of martyr in this book, I did have a lot of help along the long journey. A few of them I list below.

Peggy and Carol at AD/Parkinson's Center, Vero Beach, Florida
Annie Baez
Sandy Streeter
Dr. G. Kantzler
Dr. Deepti Sadhwani
Fran Dillon, Phyllis's sister
Natalie Shoney, Phyllis's Sister
Rick Verkamp, Phyllis's brother
George Verkamp, Phyllis's brother
CeCe Coffin, Phyllis's daughter
Jared Coffin, Phyllis's son
Todd Coffin, Phyllis's son
Briney Dillon Burley, Phyllis's niece
Connie Walsh
Louise Schmitt, PhD
Katharine Damon

Martha Eustis

Dr. Nancy Cho

Anne Douglas (Douglas Health Services, Vero Beach)

Hospice House, Vero Beach

Brenda Smith Ewers (for excellent typing, formatting, and electronic services)

And many others who visited Phyllis over the last three years of her life.

And those who sent cards of condolence and arranged for many Masses to be said in her memory. Thank you all.

CPSIA information can be obtained
at www.ICGtesting.com
Printed in the USA
BVHW03*0556050718
520865BV00004B/7/P